Body, Mind and Spirituality

Kyung Bong Koh

Body, Mind and Spirituality

A Resilience-Enhancing Approach

Springer

Kyung Bong Koh
Department of Psychiatry
Yonsei University College of Medicine
Seoul, Korea

ISBN 978-3-032-11213-2 ISBN 978-3-032-11214-9 (eBook)
https://doi.org/10.1007/978-3-032-11214-9

This Springer imprint is published by the registered company Springer Nature Switzerland AG
The registered company address is: Gewerbestrasse 11, 6330 Cham, Switzerland

Preface

Even if you are physically and mentally healthy and lack nothing, you may be in search of something because of the inner hunger and thirst you cannot fill. This is only because of your need for spirituality. When you fulfill this need, your life can be made abundant.

This book aims to help health professionals learn how to enhance resilience in patients with serious health problems (e.g., somatic symptoms and related disorders (SSRDs) and physical diseases), who are often resistant to psychosocial approaches. Furthermore, this book can help the public learn ways of increasing their resilience when faced with serious health conditions or difficult situations.

The term “resilience-enhancing approach” (REA) refers to various therapeutic modalities that enhance resilience. This approach includes biological therapy (psychopharmacotherapy and biofeedback), stress management, cognitive behavioral therapy, and spiritual approaches. Therapists should have knowledge of vulnerability, resilience, spirituality, and therapeutic modalities.

This book illustrates various clinical cases to help therapists understand how to enhance resilience in patients with SSRDs and physical diseases. Therefore, the REA is both a therapeutic and preventive intervention.

The book comprises four parts. Part I. “General Resilience-Enhancing Approaches” focuses on vulnerability and resilience, strategies for enhancing resilience, and stress management techniques. This part will help people understand the concept of resilience and promote health.

Part II. “Special Resilience-Enhancing Approaches” focuses on the cognitive behavioral approach for managing stress and for type A behavior, the role of religion and spirituality in body and mind, and ways to deal with spiritual stressors. This part emphasizes how cognitive behavioral and spiritual approaches can help enhance resilience among the general public, as well as among patients with somatic symptoms.

Part III. “Resilience-Enhancing Approaches to Somatization” includes interview techniques for managing somatizing patients and therapeutic approaches for SSRDs and chronic pain. This section mainly addresses therapeutic modalities for patients with SSRDs.

Part IV. "Resilience-Enhancing Approaches to Physical Diseases" deals with therapeutic approaches to depression and anxiety in the medically ill, functional dyspepsia, post-stroke depression, cancer, and specific cancers such as breast cancer and prostate cancer.

Herein, some of the chapters are from my previously published books, *Somatization and Psychosomatic Symptoms* (Springer, 2013) and *Stress and Somatic Symptoms: Biopsychosociospiritual Perspectives* (Springer, 2018), with a particular focus on management.

These chapters have been reorganized, shortened, and described briefly and simply for readers to understand.

This book will be of interest to both laypersons and healthcare practitioners such as psychiatrists, physicians, nurses, psychologists, and social workers dealing with stress and physical and mental health.

I thank God for enabling me to complete this work.

Seoul, Korea Kyung Bong Koh

Competing Interests The author has no competing interests to declare that are relevant to the content of this manuscript.

Contents

Part I
General Resilience-Enhancing Approaches

Chapter 1
Vulnerability and Resilience

1.1 What Is Stress?

Stress is defined as external or internal stimuli that are meaningfully perceived by a person, activate emotions, and elicit physiological changes that threaten health and survival [1]. This means that an individual's stress responses depend on his/her subjective interpretation of an event rather than the event itself [2]. Therefore, just as people perceive the same picture differently, the same event or situation may be perceived in various ways, resulting in quite different responses and outcomes—health or illness.

1.2 Causes of Stress

Major causes of stress are classified into psychosocial and environmental (bioecological) factors. This classification is based on the direct causes of the stress reaction [3].

1.2.1 Psychosocial Factors

There are four psychosocial factors: adaptation (e.g., changes in job, school, and family), frustration (e.g., prejudice and discrimination related to religion, race, sex, generation, etc.), overload (e.g., occupational, academic, and domestic), and deprivation (e.g., boredom, loneliness).

The COVID-19 pandemic can be considered a global stressor. It has brought many forms of suffering and loss. Our lives are now so intertwined with social networking

K. B. Koh, *Body, Mind and Spirituality*, https://doi.org/10.1007/978-3-032-11214-9_1

services (SNSs) that we rarely find time to relax. Modern individuals often feel lonely in crowds, leading to anxiety or panic.

1.2.2 *Environmental Factors*

These stressors include biological rhythms (e.g., disturbedsleep–wake cycles, menstruation), noise, pollution, and climate change (e.g., heat waves, cold waves, heavy rain, flooding, drought, etc.).

1.3 Stress Levels and Health

Too much stress—or too little stress (e.g., boredom)—is neither productive nor good for health [4]. Rather, optimal or moderate stress (defined as the level at which stress enhances both health and performance) can lead to a healthy and productive life [3, 4]. Paradoxically, we might say, "no stress, no happiness." The aim of stress management is not to eliminate stress entirely, but to control it so that an optimal level of arousal is maintained [4].

1.4 Background of Resilience

Stress can seriously disturb the psychological and physiological balance of an individual, but traumatic stress does not affect everyone in the same way [5]. For example, some children are capable of progressing through normal development despite exposure to significant adversity [6], although many people who experienced psychological or physical trauma during childhood remain vulnerable to a variety of mental disorders.

1.5 Differences Between Vulnerability and Resilience

Vulnerable individuals adapt poorly to stressors and exhibit inappropriate responses that may become persistent states of stress, whereas resilient individuals tend to perceive adversity as minimally threatening [5] and adapt successfully to stress, trauma, or adversity [7].

A vulnerable person can be likened to a dormant volcano that could erupt at any time—similarly, the vulnerable individual is more likely to develop disease. In contrast, a resilient person, like flowers blooming in the snow, can thrive despite adversity. Samson, a biblical figure, had tremendous physical strength but a hidden weakness in the loss of his hair. Like him, everyone has both strengths and weaknesses.

1.6 Resources for Differences Between Vulnerability and Resilience

1. Exposure to stressful events can be perceived differently by individuals [8].
2. Differences in individual vulnerability/resilience occur across sex, age, and culture [8].
3. The underlying mechanisms of vulnerability and resilience are known to depend on a combination of genetic and nongenetic factors [8].
4. Individual differences in the function of hormones, neurotransmitters, and neuropeptides may be involved in vulnerability and resilience [9].

1.7 The Relationship Between Stress and Physical Diseases

The relationship between stress and physical diseases can be illustrated as follows [10].

Stressor → cognitive appraisal → coping → psychological responses (emotional responses) → physiological responses (neuroendocrine system: hypothalamic–pituitary–adrenal (HPA) axis, sympathetic-adrenal-medullary (SAM) axis, endogenous opioids, immune system) → physical diseases.

The cerebral cortex perceives stressors and evaluates whether they are threats to the body (appraisal and reappraisal of the stressor). Individuals then select coping methods. Emotional responses—such as anxiety, depression, and anger—follow the chosen coping strategies.

Acute stressors stimulate the adrenal medulla through the sympathetic nervous system, releasing epinephrine or norepinephrine. This increases cardiac output, pulse rate, and respiratory rate, and causes metabolic changes such as alterations in blood glucose levels. However, chronic stressors activate the HPA axis, releasing cortisol, which suppresses immune function and increases the risk of physical diseases. In addition, the pituitary gland releases pro-opiomelanocortin (POMC)-induced peptides (called opioid peptides), such as endorphins, enkephalins, and dynorphins [11], which are likely to affect immune functions [12]. The endogenous opioid system is vital in regulating various physiological functions like pain relief, euphoria induction, stress resilience, cardiovascular protection, and food intake control [13].

As described above, various steps intervene in the process from stressors to disease. Cognitive appraisal and coping are two modifiable factors in this chain, playing a central role in determining vulnerability and resilience [8].

Pascal said, "Man is but a reed, but he is a thinking reed." This highlights that thought empowers individuals, even in adversity. In this context, vulnerability and resilience may depend heavily on cognitive appraisal. For example, positive reappraisal among medical students has been found to negatively correlate with stress-induced immune responses (interleukin-2) [14], suggesting that positive reappraisal enhances resilience.

An individual's cognitive appraisal and coping strategies vary, resulting in different emotional and physiological responses—and consequently, differing risks of disease.

Ineffective coping increases stress responses and can damage health. Therefore, managing stress through effective coping strategies is essential. For example, immunization activates T cells, promoting neuroprotective resilience. Stress and depression, on the other hand, suppress T-cell activity, increasing disease risk [15].

Empirical evidence supports the role of relaxation and meditation in enhancing resilience. Mediation led to a significant increase in antibody titers to the influenza vaccine compared to controls [16]. Geriatric patients who received relaxation training reported reduced distress and increased NK cell cytotoxicity, along with decreased antibody titers to latent herpes simplex virus [17]. Psychological interventions, including relaxation, improved T-cell blastogenesis in patients with breast cancer [18]. These findings suggest that relaxation and meditation are likely to promote immune function and enhance resilience.

1.8 Psychosocial Factors Associated with Vulnerability

1.8.1 Self-Perception or Self-Concept

Individuals with poor self-image, such as feelings of inferiority related to body image, academic achievement, and other personal aspects, are more vulnerable to stressors [3]. This negative self-perception can trap them in a cycle of low self-esteem ("small self") and unhappiness.

1.8.2 Personality

Type A Personality

Type A personality is characterized by an intense sense of time urgency, confidence, aggressiveness, competitiveness, ambition, and hyperactivity. These traits often elicit constant stress responses, particularly cardiovascular arousal, which may eventually lead to coronary heart disease [3]. Among these traits, competitiveness is considered one of the most significant contributors to vulnerability.

Anxious Reactive Personality

An anxious, reactive person continues to feel stress even after the stressor has passed, which can impair task performance. In particular, perfectionism increases vulnerability, as it may provoke anxiety over even minor issues [3].

1.9 Psychosocial Factors Associated with Resilience

Resilience is linked to the ability to perceive stressful events as less threatening, thereby promoting adaptive coping strategies. Such cognitive reappraisal allows individuals to re-evaluate or reframe adverse experiences in a more positive light [19].

1.9.1 Active Coping

Active coping with stress, such as engaging in problem-solving and positively reassessing aversive experiences, can help foster long-term resilience [20].

Coping by accepting the reality of stressful situations proved protective in patients with hepatitis B [21]. In an experimental study, expressing emotionally traumatic events that had not previously been disclosed to others was associated with an increased proliferative response to phytohemagglutinin (PHA) [22]. These results suggest that active coping is likely to reverse stress-induced immune responses.

In contrast, passive coping—such as denial, avoidance of conflict, and suppression of emotions—is considered ineffective because it is maladaptive and provides only short-term relief from stress [20].

1.9.2 Positive Emotions

Positive emotions (e.g., gratitude, joy) promote adaptive coping and openness to social support [23, 24], and are associated with greater cognitive flexibility and reduced autonomic activity [25].

In stressful conditions, optimism was inversely associated with stress-related interleukin-6 (IL-6) responses in healthy men, suggesting that optimism may promote resilience by counteracting stress-induced increases in inflammation [26].

1.9.3 Social Competence

Social competence, or the ability to mobilize social support, can promote resilience by fostering adaptive coping strategies [19]. For example, medical students who reported greater social support showed a stronger immune response to the hepatitis B vaccine than those with less support [27]. In addition, seeking social support was negatively associated with stress-induced immune responses (lymphocyte proliferation to PHA) in medical students [14]. In contrast, lonelier students exhibited lower NK cell activity than their less lonely peers [28]. Therefore, social competence and seeking social support are likely to enhance resilience.

1.9.4 Spirituality

Spiritual power—that is, the ability to find a sense of purpose and meaning in life in the midst of trauma—is associated with resilience [19, 29–31]. Spirituality can play a buffering role in the face of negative life events [32–36] and help enhance hope and confidence [33, 37].

1.10 Behavioral Factors Associated with Vulnerability

Preference for certain foods (e.g., those containing caffeine: coffee, tea, chocolate, and cocoa; sugar and sugar products: cake, pies, cookies, and candy; processed flour; and salt) can increase vulnerability [3]. In addition, poor coping behaviors such as unhealthy eating habits (e.g., hypoglycemia or overeating), excessive drinking and smoking, and reckless driving increase the risk of illnesses and accidents.

1.11 Behavioral Factors Associated with Resilience

Life habits (e.g., relaxation, meditation, exercise) and life satisfaction activities (e.g., humor, art, nature) can help enhance resilience. For example, relaxation and mindfulness meditation are known to improve immune responses and enhance resilience [16, 17, 38, 39]. Appreciation of nature also contributes to resilience.

1.12 Resilience and Neuroendocrine Stress Responses

Differences in the function of hormones, neurotransmitters, and neuropeptides involved in stress responses may contribute to individual differences in resilience [9].

1.12.1 Hypothalamic–Pituitary–Adrenal (HPA) Axis

Corticotropin-releasing hormone (CRH) is released by the hypothalamus in response to stress, activating the HPA axis and releasing cortisol [40]. The short-term actions of cortisol promote resilience, whereas chronic exposure to abnormally high levels of cortisol can cause immunosuppression and disease [41]. In the brain, excessive cortisol is associated with atrophic effects in the hippocampus and amygdala [42, 43], resulting in memory impairment and fear.

Resilience is associated with rapid activation of the stress response and its efficient termination [44]. Therefore, resilience may depend on the ability to constrain stress-induced increases in CRH and cortisol through a negative feedback system (e.g., relaxation) [44–46].

1.12.2 Noradrenergic System

Stress releases noradrenaline from brainstem nuclei, especially the locus coeruleus. Chronic hyper-responsiveness of the locus coeruleus is associated with anxiety disorders [47, 48], suggesting that reduced responsiveness of the locus coeruleus could promote resilience [9].

1.12.3 Serotonergic System

Serotonin modulates neural responses to stress, with both anxiogenic and anxiolytic effects depending on the brain region and receptor subtype involved [45]. Serotonin function is also closely linked to mood regulation [9]. Thus, serotonin may play an important role in resilience.

1.12.4 Dopaminergic System

Dopamine neurons are activated in response to rewards or the expectation of reward [9]. For example, pleasant experiences such as sex, shopping, eating cookies, or achieving goals can trigger dopamine release, or a "dopamine rush." This feel-good neurotransmitter is also involved in reinforcement [49], motivating individuals to repeat rewarding behaviors. In this way, dopamine can intensify positive experiences necessary for survival and help develop desirable behaviors through learning.

However, narcotic drugs such as heroin or cocaine also trigger dopamine release, leading to intense reward and potential addiction [49]. Therefore, maintaining a healthy reward system is important for enhancing resilience. Dopamine signaling facilitates fear extinction, but dopamine neurons are inhibited by aversive stimuli [9].

1.12.5 Neuropeptide Y

Neuropeptide Y (NPY) counteracts the anxiogenic effects of CRH in brain regions such as the amygdala, hippocampus, hypothalamus, and locus coeruleus. Therefore, resilience may be associated with maintaining a balance between NPY and CRH levels during stress [48].

1.13 Genetic Influences on Vulnerability and Resilience

Genetic factors affect vulnerability and resilience by influencing the balance of the autonomic nervous system—the fight-or-flight emergency reaction system. General temperament (e.g., active vs. passive, pleasant vs. unpleasant, hypersensitive vs. hyposensitive) is also partly genetically determined [50].

Genetic predisposition to high stress reactivity amplifies the effects of early-life adversity [51]. Therefore, complex interactions between an individual's genetic makeup and prior exposure to environmental stressors determine the adaptability of neurochemical stress response systems, as well as the function of neural circuits involved in stress responses [9]. For example, an individual's genetic and environmental factors, including exposure to stressors, can affect cytokine regulation, eventually leading to various diseases.

1.13.1 HPA Axis-Related Genes

Regulation of the HPA axis is affected by genetic factors. For example, polymorphisms in the CRH type 1 receptor gene (CRHR1) are known to moderate the influence of childhood abuse on adult depression, thereby exerting protective effects [52].

1.13.2 Catechol-O-Methyltransferase (COMT)-Related Genes

A genetic polymorphism (Val158Met) in the COMT gene, which encodes an enzyme that degrades dopamine (pleasure-related) and noradrenaline (anxiety-related), has been found to be associated with resilience. In contrast, the low-functioning Met158 allele can increase dopamine and noradrenaline levels, resulting in higher anxiety and reduced resilience [53].

1.13.3 Serotonin Transporter-Related Genes

The long allele of the 5-HTTLPR gene, involved in mood regulation, has been associated with emotional resilience [54]. However, carriers of the short allele of 5-HTTLPR appear to be at increased risk for depression when exposed to stressful life events, compared with long-allele homozygotes in some studies [55–57].

1.13.4 NPY-Related Genes

Higher levels of NPY mRNA (messenger RNA) expression, associated with lower anxiety and pain suppression, are likely to enhance resilience [58].

1.14 Gene–Gene and Gene–Environment Interactions

Gene–gene and gene–environment interactions may contribute to individual differences in stress responses.

1.14.1 Gene–Gene Interactions

For example, an interaction between monoamine oxidase A (MAOA) and COMT genes affects endocrine responses to psychological challenge tasks [59], thereby negatively influencing resilience.

1.14.2 Gene–Environment Interactions

For example, an interaction among 5-HTTLPR, COMT, and stressful life events has been shown to affect the risk of depression [60], thereby negatively influencing resilience.

1.15 Epigenetic Mechanisms of Vulnerability and Resilience

Epigenetics refers to processes that induce heritable changes in gene expression without altering the DNA sequence itself. These mechanisms occur primarily at the chromatin level and often involve DNA methylation. Epigenetic mechanisms are known to play important roles in gene–environment interactions that affect stress responses [8]. They can be influenced by environmental factors such as diet, culture, and stress [61–63].

Epigenetic changes can cause lifelong differences in behavior [64]. For example, memes—sociocultural elements such as culture-related knowledge, information, and behaviors—can be transmitted across generations through imitation, thereby affecting resilience. Some endemic memes are introduced into the minds of children from early life and may be either protective or pathogenic [65].

1.16 Neural Circuitry of Resilience

Understanding the neural circuitry involved in fear, reward, emotional regulation, and social behavior is essential for exploring resilience. Studies on the neural regulation of endocrine and autonomic responses to stress can be conducted in humans by monitoring stress responses during functional imaging studies [66].

1.16.1 Neural Circuitry of Fear

Brain imaging studies in healthy participants have shown that the amygdala is involved in the acquisition of fear conditioning [67], while the extinction of fear memory involves both the ventromedial prefrontal cortex (vmPFC) and the amygdala [67, 68]. In particular, the vmPFC appears to mediate the shifting of fear to a different stimulus under stressful conditions [69]. Thus, the neural circuitry of fear plays an important role in resilience.

1.16.2 Neural Circuitry of Reward

In fMRI (functional magnetic resonance imaging) studies, patients with major depressive disorder and posttraumatic stress disorder (PTSD) have shown reduced striatal activation during reward-related tasks. These findings suggest dysfunction in the reward system in these patients [70–72]. Trait optimism is linked to reward circuit function; specifically, activation in the rostral anterior cingulate cortex (rACC) is positively associated with optimism [73]. Therefore, optimism, through its connection to reward circuit function, is likely to enhance resilience.

1.16.3 Neural Circuitry of Emotional Regulation

A greater capacity for emotional regulation has been associated with stress resilience [74]. fMRI studies [75, 76] suggest that the prefrontal cortex (PFC) regulates the intensity of emotional responses (e.g., fear and anxiety) by modulating amygdala activation. Thus, emotional regulation can be supported by both the stabilization of the amygdala (e.g., via relaxation) and the strengthening of the PFC.

1.16.4 Neural Circuits of Social Behavior

Social competence and openness to social support are core characteristics of resilient individuals [9]. In particular, the capacity for empathy enables individuals to generate appropriate emotional responses in social contexts and may be related to social competence [77, 78].

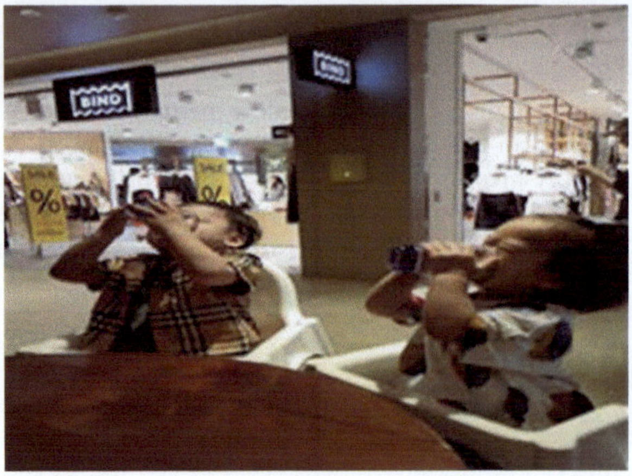

Fig. 1.1 A younger infant is imitating another infant's performance

Mirror Neuron System

Experimentally, cortical neurons are similarly activated both when an animal performs a task and when it observes the same task performed by another [79]. These neurons "mirror" the behavior of the other, as though the observer were itself acting. This is referred to as the *mirror neuron system.* In addition, mirror neurons were found to be similarly activated when a newborn monkey observed and then imitated a human's tongue protrusion [80]. This system, acting in conjunction with limbic brain regions, likely plays a central role in empathy—that is, understanding others' emotions and intentions [78].

If this mirror neuron system exists in humans, its activation is expected to enhance resilience by supporting empathy and learning through imitation (Fig. 1.1).

Activation of the VmPFC

The vmPFC is activated both when people think about their own mental states and when they consider the mental states of others. Lesions in this region are associated with impairments in social emotions such as shame, guilt, and empathy [81].

Oxytocin

The neuropeptide oxytocin appears to facilitate social attachment by improving a person's ability to infer the mental states of others. It also reduces amygdala activation in response to fear-inducing visual stimuli [82, 83]. Imaging studies show that mutual cooperation induces activation in reward circuitry regions, which are modulated by oxytocin [84]. Thus, oxytocin is likely to enhance resilience.

Love and Neural Responses to Threat

In an fMRI study of married women, holding hands with their husbands decreased neural responses to the threat of receiving a shock, and this effect was proportional to the quality of their relationship [85]. This finding suggests that love can play a key role in promoting resilience.

1.17 An Integrated Aspect of the Neural Circuitry Related to Resilience

Taken together, adaptive functioning of the neural circuits involved in fear, emotional regulation, and social behavior can help enhance resilience by increasing an individual's capacity to face fears, experience positive emotions, reframe stressful events positively, and seek social support. Thus, resilience is an active process—not merely the absence of pathology—and can be promoted by enhancing protective factors [9].

1.18 Biopsychosocial Model of Resilience

The biopsychosocial model of resilience [86] can be summarized as follows:

Psychological factors such as self-efficacy, optimism, positive emotions, and cognitive reappraisal directly affect resilience. These psychological factors interact with the neural circuitry and stress response system, thereby influencing resilience.

Genetic, epigenetic, and environmental factors (e.g., resources, family, and community support) also affect the neural circuitry and stress response system, contributing to resilience.

Therapeutic and preventive interventions (e.g., practicing cognitive reappraisal) can enhance resilience by influencing biopsychosocial factors—including the neural circuitry and stress response system; psychological traits such as self-efficacy, optimism, positive emotions, and cognitive reappraisal; and environmental supports.

1.19 Summary

1. Psychological factors such as self-efficacy, optimism, positive emotions, and cognitive reappraisal directly affect resilience. These factors interact with the neural circuitry and stress response system.
2. Genetic, epigenetic, and environmental factors (e.g., resources, family, and community support) influence the neural circuitry and stress response system, thereby enhancing resilience.

3. Therapeutic and preventive interventions such as stress management, cognitive behavioral therapy, prayer, and psychopharmacotherapy can enhance resilience by targeting biopsychosocial factors.
4. Spiritual power—that is, the ability to find purpose and meaning in life amid trauma—is associated with resilience.
5. Beyond the personal level, greater unity and collaboration are needed to combat shared challenges such as pandemics, climate change, and pollution, thereby promoting social and global resilience.

References

1. Lipowski, Z. J. (1985). *Psychosomatic medicine and liaison psychiatry.* Plenum Medical Book Co.
2. Reiser, M. F. (1984). Psychophysiology of stress and its sequelae. In M. F. Reiser (Ed.), *Mind, brain, body: Toward a convergence of psychoanalysis and neurobiology.* Basic Books.
3. Girdano, D. A., & Everly, G. (1979). *Controlling stress and tension: A holistic approach.* Prentice-Hall.
4. Rice, P. L. (1987). *Stress and health: Principles and practice for coping and wellness.* Brooks/Cole Publishing.
5. Del Giudice, M., Ellis, B. J., & Shirtcliff, E. A. (2011). The adaptive calibration model of stress responsivity. *Neuroscience and Biobehavioral Reviews, 35*, 1562–1592.
6. Masten, A. S. (2001). Ordinary magic. Resilience processes in development. *American Psychologist, 56*, 227–238.
7. Rutter, M. (2006). Implications of resilience concepts for scientific understanding. *Annals. New York Academy of Sciences, 1094*, 1–12.
8. Franklin, T. B., Saab, B. J., & Mansuy, I. M. (2012). Neural mechanisms of stress resilience and vulnerability. *Neuron, 75*, 747–761.
9. Feder, A., Nestler, E. J., & Charney, D. S. (2009). Psychobiology and molecular genetics of resilience. *Nature Reviews Neuroscience, 10*, 446–457.
10. Koh, K. B. (2018). *Stress and somatic symptoms: Biopsychosociospiritual perspectives.* Springer.
11. Peciña, M., Karp, J. F., Mathew, S., et al. (2019). Endogenous opioid system dysregulation in depression: Implications for new therapeutic approaches. *Molecular Psychiatry, 24*, 576–587.
12. Fawzy, F. I. (1995). Behavior and immunity. In H. I. Kaplan & B. J. Sadock (Eds.), *Comprehensive textbook of psychiatry*. Williams & Wilkins.
13. Froehlich, J. C. (1997). Opioid peptides. *Alcohol Health and Research World, 21*, 132–136.
14. Koh, K. B., Choe, E., Song, J. E., et al. (2006). Effect of coping on endocrinoimmune functions in different stress situations. *Psychiatry Research, 143*, 223–234.
15. Miller, A. H. (2010). Depression and immunity: A role for T cells? *Brain, Behavior, and Immunity, 24*, 1–8.
16. Davidson, R. J., Kabat-zinn, J., Schumacher, J., et al. (2003). Alterations in brain and immune function produced by mindfulness meditation. *Psychosomatic Medicine, 65*, 564–570.
17. Kiecolt-Glaser, J. K., Glaser, R., & Williger, D. (1985). Psychosocial enhancement of immunocompetence in a geriatric population. *Health Psychology, 4*, 25–41.
18. Andersen, B. L., Golden-Kreutz, D., Emery, C. F., et al. (2007). Distress reduction from a psychological intervention contributes to improved health for cancer patients. *Brain, Behavior, and Immunity, 21*, 953–961.
19. Southwick, S. M., Vythilingam, M., & Charney, D. S. (2005). The psychobiology of depression and resilience to stress: Implications for prevention and treatment. *Annual Review of Clinical Psychology, 1*, 255–291.

20. Sherrer, M. V. (2011). The role of cognitive appraisal in adaptation to traumatic stress in adults with serious mental illness: A critical review. *Trauma, Violence & Abuse, 12*, 151–167.
21. Burns, V. E., Carroll, D., Ring, C., et al. (2002). Stress, coping, and hepatitis B antibody status. *Psychosomatic Medicine, 64*, 287–293.
22. Fawzy, F. I. (1995). Behavior and immunity. In H. I. Kaplan & B. J. Sodock (Eds.), *Comprehensive textbook of psychiatry*. Willams & Wilkins.
23. Ong, A. D., Bergeman, C. S., Bisconti, T. L., et al. (2006). Psychological resilience, positive emotions, and successful adaptation to stress in later life. *Journal of Personality and Social Psychology, 91*, 730–749.
24. Tugade, M. M., & Fredrickson, B. L. (2004). Resilient individuals use positive emotions to bounce back from negative emotional experiences. *Journal of Personality and Social Psychology, 86*, 320–333.
25. Fredrickson, B. L. (2001). The role of positive emotions in positive psychology. The broaden-and-build theory of positive emotions. *American Psychologist, 56*, 218–226.
26. Brydon, L., Walker, C., Wawrzyniak, A. J., et al. (2009). Dispositional optimism and stress-induced changes in immunity and negative mood. *Brain, Behavior, and Immunity, 23*, 810–816.
27. Glaser, R., Kiecolt-Glaser, J. K., Bonneau, R., et al. (1992). Stress-induced modulation of the immune response to recombinant hepatitis B vaccine. *Psychosomatic Medicine, 54*, 22–29.
28. Kiecolt-Glaser, J. K., Garner, W., Speicher, C., et al. (1984). Psychosocial modifiers of immunocompetence in medical students. *Psychosomatic Medicine, 46*, 7–14.
29. Alim, T. N., Feder, A., Graves, R. E., et al. (2008). Trauma, resilience, and recovery in a high-risk African-American population. *American Journal of Psychiatry, 165*, 1566–1575.
30. Ryff, C. D., & Keyes, C. L. (1995). The structure of psychological well-being revisited. *Journal of Personality and Social Psychology, 69*, 719–727.
31. Pargement, K. I., Koenig, B. W., & Perez, L. (1998). Patterns of positive and negative religious coping with major life stressors. *Journal of Scientific Study of Religion, 37*, 710–724.
32. Crawford, M., Handal, P., & Weiner, R. (1989). The relationship between religion and mental health/distress. *Review of Religious Research, 31*, 16–22.
33. Ellison, C. (1991). Religious involvement and subjective well-being. *Journal of Health and Social Behavior, 32*, 80–99.
34. Hathaway, W., & Pargament, K. (1990). Intrinsic religiousness, religious coping, and psychosocial competence: A covariance structural anaylsis. *Journal of Scientific Study of Religion, 29*, 423–441.
35. Pargament, K., Kennell, J., Hathaway, W., et al. (1988). Religion and the problem-solving process: Three styles of coping. *Journal of Scientific Study of Religion, 27*, 90–104.
36. Ross, C. (1990). Religion and psychological distress. *Journal of Scientific Study of Religion, 29*, 235–245.
37. Maton, R. (1987). Spiritual discernment in psychiatric patients. *Journal of Religion and Health, 26*, 125–130.
38. Green, R. G., & Green, M. L. (1987). Relaxation increases salivary immunoglobulin A. *Psychological Reports, 61*, 623–629.
39. Koh, K. B., Lee, Y., Beyn, K. M., et al. (2008). Counter-stress effects of relaxation on proinflammatory and anti-inflammatory cytokines. *Brain, Behavior, and Immunity, 22*, 1130–1137.
40. Heim, C., & Nemeroff, C. B. (2001). The role of childhood trauma in the neurobiology of mood and anxiety disorders: Preclinical and clinical studies. *Biological Psychiatry, 49*, 1023–1039.
41. Karlamangla, A. S., Singer, B. H., McEwen, B. S., et al. (2002). Allostatic load as a predictor of functional decline. MacArthur studies of successful aging. *Journal of Clinical Epidemiology, 55*, 696–710.
42. McEwen, B. S., & Milner, T. A. (2007). Hippocampal formation: Shedding light on the influence of sex and stress on the brain. *Brain Research Reviews, 55*, 343–355.
43. Brown, E. S., Woolston, D. J., & Frol, A. B. (2008). Amygdala volume in patients receiving chronic corticosteroid therapy. *Biological Psychiatry, 63*, 705–709.

44. de Kloet, E. R., Joels, M., & Holsboer, F. (2005). Stress and the brain: From adaptation to disease. *Nature Reviews Neuroscience, 6*, 463–475.
45. Charney, D. S. (2004). Psychobiological mechanisms of resilience and vulnerability: Implications for successful adaptation to extreme stress. *American Journal of Psychiatry, 161*, 195–216.
46. de Kloet, E. R., Deriik, R. H., & Meijer, O. C. (2007). Therapy insight: Is there an imbalanced response of meineralocorticoid and glucocorticoic receptors in depression? *Nature Clinical Practice Endocrinology & Metabolism, 3*, 168–179.
47. Charney, D. S. (2003). Neuroanatomical circuits modulating fear and anxiety behaviors. *Acta Psychiatrica Scandinavica. Supplementum, 417*, 38–50.
48. Sajdyk, T. J., Shekhar, A., & Gehlert, D. R. (2004). Interactions between NPY and CRF in the amygdala to regulate emotionality. *Neuropeptides, 38*, 225–234.
49. Watson, S. (2024, April 18). *Dopamine: The pathway to pleasure*. Harvard Health Publishing. www.health.harvard.edu
50. Fuller, J. L., & Thompson, W. R. (1978). *Foundations of behavior genetics*. Mosby.
51. McIlwrick, S., Rechenberg, A., Matthes, M., et al. (2016). Genetic predisposition for high stress reactivity amplifies effects of early-life adversity. *Psychoneuroendocrinology, 70*, 85–97.
52. Bradley, R. G., Binder, E. B., Epstein, M. P., et al. (2008). Influence of child abuse on adult depression: Moderation by the corticotropin-releasing hormone receptor gene. *Archives of General Psychiatry, 65*, 190–200.
53. Heinz, A., & Smolka, M. N. (2006). The effects of catechol O-methyltransferase genotype on brain activation elicited by affective stimuli and cognitive tasks. *Reviews in the Neurosciences, 17*, 359–367.
54. Stein, M. B., Campbell-Sills, L., & Gelernter, J. (2009). Genetic variation in 5-HTTLPR is associated with emotional resilience. *American Journal of Medical Genetics. Part B, Neuropsychiatric Genetics, 150B*, 900–906.
55. Caspi, A., Sugden, K., Moffitt, T. E., et al. (2003). Influence of life stress on depression: Moderation by a polymorphism in the 5-HTT gene. *Science, 301*, 386–389.
56. Kendler, K. S., Kuhn, J. W., Vittum, J., et al. (2005). The interaction of stressful life events and a serotonin transporter polymorphism in the prediction of episodes of major depression: A replication. *Archives of General Psychiatry, 62*, 529–535.
57. Gillespie, N. A., Whitfield, J. B., Williams, B., et al. (2005). The relationship between stressful life events, the serotonin transporter (5-HTTLPR) genotype and major depression. *Psychological Medicine, 35*, 101–111.
58. Zhou, Z., Zhu, G., Hariri, A. R., et al. (2008). Genetic variation in human NPY expression affects stress response and emotion. *Nature, 452*, 997–1001.
59. Jabbi, M., Korf, J., Kema, I. P., et al. (2007). Convergent genetic modulation of the endocrine stress response involves polymorphic variations of 5-HTT, COMT and MAOA. *Molecular Psychiatry, 12*, 483–490.
60. Mandelli, L., Serretti, A., Marino, E., et al. (2007). Interaction between serotonin transporter gene, catechol-O-methyltransferase gene and stressful life events in mood disorders. *International Journal of Neuropsychopharmacology, 10*, 437–447.
61. Franklin, T. B., & Mansuy, I. M. (2011). The involvement of epigenetic defects in mental retardation. *Neurobiology of Learning and Memory, 96*, 61–67.
62. Kubota, T., Miyake, K., & Hirasawa, T. (2012). Epigenetic understanding of gene-environment interactions in psychiatric disorders: A new concept of clinical genetics. *Clinical Epigenetics, 4*, 1.
63. McEwen, B. S., Eiland, L., Hunter, R. G., et al. (2012). Stress and anxiety: Structural plasticity and epigenetic regulation as a consequence of stress. *Neuropharmacology, 62*, 3–12.
64. Krishnan, V., Han, M.-H., Graham, D. L., et al. (2007). Molecular adaptations underlying susceptibility and resistance to social defeat in brain reward regions. *Cell, 131*, 391–404.
65. Leigh, H. (2013). Genes, memes, culture, and psychosomatic medicine: An integrative model. In K. B. Koh (Ed.), *Somatization and psychosomatic symptoms*. Springer.

66. Dedovic, K., Renwick, R., Najmeh, K. M., et al. (2005). The montreal imaging stress task: Using functional imaging to investigate the effects of perceiving and processing psychosocial stress in the human brain. *Journal of Psychiatry and Neuroscience, 30*, 319–325.
67. Delgado, M. R., Olsson, A., & Phelps, E. A. (2006). Extending animal models of fear conditioning to humans. *Biological Psychology, 73*, 39–48.
68. Milad, M. R., Quinn, B. T., Pitman, R. K., et al. (2005). Thickness of ventromedial prefrontal cortex in humans is correlated with extinction memory. *Proceedings of the National academy of Sciences of the United States of America, 102*, 10706–10711.
69. Schiller, D., Levy, I., Niv, Y., et al. (2008). From fear to safety and back: Reversal of fear in the human brain. *Journal of Neuroscience, 28*, 11517–11525.
70. Pizzagalli, D. A., Holmes, A. J., Dillon, D. J., et al. (2008). Reduced caudate and nucleus accumbens response to rewards in unmedicated subjects with major depressive disorder. *American Journal of Psychiatry, 166*, 702–710.
71. Sailer, U., Robinson, S., Fischmeister, F., et al. (2008). Altered reward processing in the nucleus accumbens and mesial prefrontal cortex of patients with posttraumatic stress disorder. *Neuropsychologia, 46*, 2836–2844.
72. Drevets, W. C., Price, J. L., & Furey, M. L. (2008). Brain structural and functional abnormalties in mood disorders: Implication for neurocircuitry models of depression. *Brain Structure & Function, 213*, 93–118.
73. Sharot, T., Riccardi, A. M., Raio, C. M., et al. (2007). Neural mechanisms mediating optimism bias. *Nature, 450*, 102–105.
74. Ressler, K. J., & Mayberg, H. S. (2007). Targeting abnormal neural circuits in mood and anxiety disorders: From the laboratory to the clinic. *Nature Neuroscience, 10*, 1116–1124.
75. Goldin, P. R., McRae, K., Ramel, W., et al. (2008). The neural bases of emotion regulation: Reappraisal and suppression of negative emotion. *Biological Psychiatry, 63*, 577–586.
76. Ochsner, K. N., Ray, R. D., Cooper, J. C., et al. (2004). For better or for worse: Neural systems supporting the cognitive down- and up-regulation of negative emotion. *NeuroImage, 23*, 483–499.
77. Iarocci, G., Yager, J., & Elfers, T. (2007). What gene-environment interactions can tell us about social competence in typical and atypical populations. *Brain and Cognition, 65*, 112–117.
78. Storm, E. E., & Tecott, L. H. (2005). Social circuits: Peptidergic regulation of mammalian social behavior. *Neuron, 47*, 483–486.
79. Rizzolatti, G., & Craighero, L. (2004). The mirror-neuron system. *Annual Review of Neuroscience, 27*, 169–192.
80. Ferrari, P. F., Visalberghi, E., Paukner, A., et al. (2006). Neonatal imitation in rhesus macaques. *PLoS Biology, 4*(9), e302. https://doi.org/10.1371/journal.pbio.0040302.
81. Pfeifer, J. H., Iacoboni, M., Mazziotta, J. C., et al. (2008). Mirroring others' emotions relates to empathy and interpersonal competence in children. *NeuroImage, 39*, 2067–2085.
82. Domes, G., Heinrichs, M., Michel, A., et al. (2007). Oxytocin improves mind-reading in humans. *Biological Psychiatry, 61*, 731–733.
83. Radke, S., Volman, I., Kokal, I., et al. (2017). Oxytocin reduces amygdala responses during threat approach. *Psychoneuroendocrinology, 79*, 160–166.
84. Rilling, J. K., Gutman, D. A., Zeh, T. R., et al. (2002). A neural basis for social cooperation. *Neuron, 35*, 395–405.
85. Coan, J. A., Schaefer, H. S., & Davidson, R. J. (2006). Lending a hand: Social regulation of the neural response to threat. *Psychological Science, 17*, 1032–1039.
86. Feder, A., Fred-Torres, S., Southwick, S. M., et al. (2019). The biology of human resilience: Opportunities for enhancing resilience across the life span. *Biological Psychiatry, 86*, 443–453.

Chapter 2
Strategies for Enhancing Resilience

2.1 What Is Resilience-Enhancing Approach?

Resilience-enhancing approach (REA) refers to a variety of therapeutic modalities that enhance resilience and is also referred to as the biopsychosociospiritual approach. This approach includes biological therapy (psychopharmacotherapy and biofeedback), stress management, cognitive behavioral therapy, and spiritual approaches. Therefore, therapists should have the knowledge regarding vulnerabilities, resilience, spirituality, and therapeutic modalities.

Therapists can play the role of a guide, teacher, and listener to help patients enhance their resilience so that they can cope with the stress and adversities they face in life. In addition, REA is expected to improve the quality of life as well as symptoms of the patients. REA is not only a therapeutic intervention but also a preventive one. In this respect, REA can be applied to the general public as well as to patients, especially those with somatization and physical diseases.

2.2 It Is Crucial to Know One's Constitution

Similar to appearances, the concentration of biochemicals in blood varies from person to person. This is because people are born with different constitutions. For example, some babies cannot feed on mother's milk right from birth because they congenitally lack lactase, an enzyme that breaks down lactose, a sugar present in milk and other dairy products [2]. Even later in life, they cannot digest milk or milk products (e.g., cheese, yogurt, bread, etc.) as this may cause diarrhea and abdominal pain [1].

It might take a long time for people to recognize their weak constitution, which can cause immense suffering. Similarly, some people may be born with a genetic deficiency of alcohol dehydrogenase (ALDH2 gene: rs671 allele), making it difficult to metabolize alcohol [3]. They are likely to experience facial flushing, headaches,

K. B. Koh, *Body, Mind and Spirituality*, https://doi.org/10.1007/978-3-032-11214-9_2

tachycardia, and nausea on consuming alcohol [4]. Nonetheless, they may like to drink alcohol, and continue to drink, resulting in interpersonal conflicts and black-outs (a sudden loss of memory), often ending up in psychiatric departments for treatment. Such individuals should avoid drinking alcohol because they do not have the capability to effectively metabolize acetaldehyde, a toxic byproduct of alcohol metabolism [3], similar to people who are allergic to certain foods (e.g., fish).

Depression is another example. Some people may be temporarily depressed by stressors, whereas others may be genetically depressed [5, 6] due to a genetic deficiency of neurotransmitters related to depression (e.g., serotonin) [7–9]. This can be clarified by considering the family history of people with depression. In particular, if one continues to be in depression despite the alleviation of stressors, one is likely to be constitutionally depressed. In such cases, antidepressants must be administered continually to replenish the deficient serotonin neurotransmitters. Moreover, as it takes 2–4 weeks for antidepressants to show effect [10, 11], keeping the medication level constant in the body is important. Discontinuing medications, even temporarily, before at least six months of treatment may predispose such individuals to a high risk of depression recurrence [12]. In such cases, individuals should consult a psychiatrist to choose an antidepressant appropriate for them; that is, one with fewer side effects and better therapeutic effects.

Importantly, one needs to accept their genetic predisposition and avoid foods (e.g., milk or milk products) or drinks (e.g., alcohol) that may trigger issues. In cases with a genetic predisposition to depression, continual use of antidepressants such as selective serotonin reuptake inhibitors (SSRIs) may be necessary. However, it is also essential to learn how to address and overcome other (nongenetic) factors, such as problems with daily habits, interpersonal relationships, and environmental adaptation. Thus, differentiating between the two helps enhance resilience.

2.3 Changes in the Body Signal Stress

Stress is an integral part of living. Too much stress—or too little stress—is neither productive nor good for health. In this respect, maintaining moderate stress is the secret to good health [13]. Therefore, identifying if one is experiencing stress is important. One may feel angry, anxious, or depressed and think, "I am stressed." Otherwise, it might not be easy to recognize whether one is under stress. However, one way to recognize stress is through changes in one's body [14]. These changes in the body in response to stress may vary from person to person. For example, change in body weight may be an indicator of perceived stress, as may be a sense of heaviness in the head or headaches, fatigue, indigestion, etc. Once an individual recognizes the symptoms, they must stop doing what they are doing and begin to practice relaxation. The habit of listening to even the smallest changes in one's body can prevent serious diseases [15].

2.4 Positive Thinking Helps in Maintaining Good Health

The so-called happiness and unhappiness depend on our minds, rather than on actual situations. There may be something good and bad in anything; the consequences vary in how one thinks. Optimism (positive thinking) is associated with a healthy lipid profile, including lower triglyceride and cholesterol (LDL cholesterol) levels [16] and higher HDL cholesterol levels [17]. Additionally, it boosts immunity and reduces the risk of cardiovascular diseases and cancer [18]. In contrast, pessimism (negative thinking) is associated with cardiovascular mortality [19]. Regardless of how difficult one's situation is, a hole can actually be seen by those who believe that there is a hole for one's survival. Among the Jews who were locked up in a concentration camp, the survivors were found to be those who tried to live with a positive meaning in life [20].

2.5 Repetition of Words or Behaviors Enhances Resilience [15]

Resilience may be the result of the repetitive practice of certain words and behaviors. To become optimistic, one should learn to think and act optimistically. Most people who overcome disabilities or difficult times are optimistic. These people bounce back like a roly poly even if they fail. The Korean boxer, Soowhan Hong, who won the championship in Panama in 1977, was knocked down four times in the second round, but came back to knock out his opponent in the third round. Later, he recalled, saying, "I threw a punch reflexively but not consciously." His victory was the result of repetitive practice performed as usual.

Some people can change their behavior. For example, a professor at a medical school quit his job to study theology, while a successful businessman joined a temple to become a monk and engaged in Zen meditation. This was because the framework of their personal beliefs changed.

They realized that the value of life does not depend only on money, knowledge, or honor. In other words, they found greater value in their callings, such as introspection, self-discovery, or seeking spirituality, than in what they had sought earlier. Such a framework of thinking can have a great influence on one's behavior compared to others.

First, one must observe what one says or how one behaves repetitively, and then think about which framework of thinking is influencing one's words and behaviors. This will help in accessing the problems one is facing more deeply. Thereafter, one must ask oneself whether what one says or does then is what one really wants to do; else, one may need to change something. If one needs to make some changes, one must find a greater framework (e.g., contribution to society) for one's thinking compared to a more restricted one (e.g., personal needs).

2.6 Look at the Whole Rather Than the Parts

People may lose many other important things when trying to scramble for only gains. Drawing on a quotation often attributed to Thomas Huxley, we can say that sometimes we should know "something about everything" but sometimes "everything about something." This statement highlights "the benefits of both general and specific knowledge."

Trying to fix only the wrong part instead of looking at the whole may lead to wastage of both time and money. Many large accidents happen when problems are temporarily and seemingly managed rather than fundamentally solved. One may have a difficult time when one only sees the problem in parts and not as a whole. For example, a woman in her late 40s resented the way her mother treated her, saying, "Mom made me work, not my younger sister," "Mom scolded me for getting home late once at night, not my sister." She even thought of her mother as a stepmother. Feeling discriminated against by her mother, she attempted suicide by taking dozens of medications. After marriage, however, she came to understand her mother's behavior to some degree. She learned that her mother had wanted her to set a good example for her sister. Sometimes, having the habit of reviewing what we have done or felt as a whole can help prevent us from making big mistakes [15].

2.7 Work Means Health, While Growth Means Happiness

I empathized with Hyung Suck Kim, a 104-year-old professor emeritus, when he said in his lecture: "Work refers to health, while growth refers to happiness." One is told to exercise for health, but working is not any less important than exercise to keep one healthy. Without working, one is likely to feel depressed and futile. Therefore, those who do not work after retirement often look older than those who do.

A man in his 50s quit his long-term job to rest because he had given too much to his company. He had no financial problems because he made a fortune, and all of his children had graduated from college. Initially, he was satisfied with quitting his job, feeling lighter and more relaxed than when he was working. However, after two months, he did not feel the same pleasure in playing golf, which he enjoyed; rather, he felt empty and tired, casting doubt on the meaning of life. He began to feel regret over quitting his job in haste. Later, he got a new job despite a lower pay than before his retirement, and regained his vigor, saying, "I feel like I am living a new life."

When we grow old and learn what we have always wanted to or what we could not learn till now, we feel happy. In my case, I sometimes spent time doing nothing during the COVID-19 pandemic, like a squirrel going round in a treadwheel. My wife proposed participating in a play, and I agreed as I needed some stimulus. This time, however, we were supposed to perform a musical instead of a play, and it required considerable singing on my part. I was confident in performing in a play because I had participated in worship dramas several times in the church since I retired, but it was a great burden for me to learn to sing. Nevertheless, I persistently practiced singing songs, as I decided to take advantage of this opportunity to learn to sing. The harder I practiced, the better I felt. I could complete the musical performance five times successfully. Thereafter, I participated in another musical performance and was happy to discover that I had performed better than before.

2.8 Living with a Sense of Minor Inadequacies [15]

People tend to work less when they feel they lack nothing. Instead of working, they are likely to be lazy and indulge in drinking, gambling, or using drugs such as marijuana. Among those who suddenly became rich when the price of their land soared in the southern areas of Seoul, Korea, some visited the Department of Psychiatry with the problem of alcohol abuse. They did not find pleasure in anything other than drinking alcohol, because they no longer needed to work.

Long ago, I was very impressed by Bertrand Russell's words written on a large signboard on the way to the Boston airport: "To be without some of the things you want is an indispensable part of happiness."

We work hard to fill up something when we feel inadequate. We also seek safety when anxious. Such individuals tend to work extensively and are more likely to succeed.

One loses the taste of food when one eats too much, regardless of how delicious it is. Likewise, one loses the pleasures of life when one has everything. Adler, a psychoanalyst, said, "everyone is born with a sense of inferiority." Ultimately, getting over such a sense of inferiority ahead of others leads to success and happiness.

2.9 Self-Control, Rather Than Freedom, Can Help Maintain Good Health [15]

Balancing freedom and self-control can help maintain good health. However, people tend to acquire as much freedom as they possibly can. There arises the need for self-control. Those who eat too much are likely to have stomach problems. Heavy drinking can ruin both the body and mind. Overspending can impact one's household economy and lead to bankruptcy. Those who were poor during their childhood and could not do what they had wanted tend to allow their children to have their own way when they have earned sufficient money. In such situations, it is not easy for children to live and behave moderately because they enjoy the freedom but have not learned about self-control.

A college professor allowed his children to enjoy as much freedom as possible. Consequently, his daughter lost her self-control in relationships with the opposite gender during her college life, sometimes used hallucinogens, and frequently indulged in drinking and smoking; her marriage eventually ended in a divorce. By contrast, well-disciplined children often grow well and live up to their parents' expectations.

2.10 People in Sync with Nature Are Strong [15]

While serving in the army, once on my way to the bachelor officers' quarters (BOQ), looking up at the star-studded sky, smelling the grass, hearing the wind whistling and insects chirping, I was enthralled by the mystery of the universe, and suddenly felt like God was nearby. Such experiences reminded me of the mystery of nature.

Sometimes, getting out of a busy city and going to the mountains, seeing the forests and trees, and hearing the sounds of water and birds singing can make us calm. Reflecting on the mystery of nature refreshes one's body and mind and offers an opportunity to look deeper into one's mind and far into the future. It also deepens one's thinking and expands one's horizons.

2.11 Be Empty and Fill Up [15]

Please be empty and then fill up to maintain mental and physical health.

As we know from our experiences, our brain and mind need to be empty to deal with all the unpleasantness that we encounter; otherwise, we would be vulnerable to stressors, resulting in short temper and explosive outbursts. We need to train ourselves to react positively to any stimulus by emptying the brain and mind through rest, exercise, meditation, and self-control, and by filling them up with positive thinking and words. This will allow us to cope well even in difficult situations.

2.12 Manage Stress with STRESS

Long ago, I was extremely impressed by a sermon preached by the reverend of the Crystal Church, Robert Schuller, on television. His sermon was about STRESS; the acronym stood for spiritual power, think positively, rest, exercise, seek good things you can do, and scripture. He used this acronym to inform us of ways to manage stress [15].

Spirituality can give us the power to overcome the difficult things we face while doing good things (God's work), for God is always with us. The fruits of the Spirit are love, joy, peace, patience, kindness, goodness, faithfulness, gentleness, and self-control (Galatians 5:22, 23). Among them, self-control can be seen as an element that many people today need most desperately to maintain their health. However, despite being physically and mentally healthy and lacking nothing, one may still be searching for something. This search is due to an inner hunger or thirst one is unable to fill. This is the need for spirituality.

The World Health Organization (WHO) defines health as "a state of complete physical, mental, and social wellbeing." In 1986, the concept of health expanded beyond the absence of disease [21]. In this regard, spirituality can also help promote health [22–24], resulting in a change in quality of life.

2.13 Summary

1. Resilience-enhancing approach (REA) refers to a variety of therapeutic modalities that enhance resilience; hence, it is also known as the biopsychosociospiritual approach. This approach includes biological therapy (psychopharmacotherapy and biofeedback), stress management, cognitive behavioral therapy, and spiritual approaches.
2. As general strategies for enhancing resilience, it is crucial to recognize the constitution of and changes in one's body; to look at the whole rather than the parts; to recognize that working means being healthy, while growth means happiness; to empty the brain and the mind and fill them up; and to manage stress using STRESS.
3. Positive thinking, the repetition of words or behaviors, a sense of minor inadequacies, self-control, and a nature-friendly attitude can help enhance resilience.

References

1. Di Stenfano, M., Miceli, E., Mazzocchi, S., et al. (2007). Visceral hypersensitivity and intolerance symptoms in lactose malabsorption. *Neurogastroenterology and Motility, 19*(11), 887–895.
2. Kuokkanen, M., Kokkonen, J., Enttah, N. S., et al. (2006). Translated region of the lactase gene underlie congenital lactase deficiency. *American Journal of Human Genetics, 78*, 339–344.
3. Chen, Y. C., Peng, G. S., Wang, M. F., et al. (2009). Polymorphism of ethanol—Metabolism genes and alcoholism: Correlation of allelic variations with the pharmacokinetic and pharmacodynamic consequences. *Chemico-Biological Interactions, 178*, 2–7.
4. Harada, S., Agarwal, D. P., Goedde, H. W. (1981). Aldehyde dehydrogenase deficiency as cause of facial flushing reaction to alcohol in Japanese. *Lancet, 2*(8253), 982.
5. Kendler, K. S. (1998). Major depression and the environment: A psychiatric genetic perspective. *Pharmaco Psychiatry, 31*, 5–9.
6. Malhi, G. S., Moore, J., & McGuffin, P. (2000). The genetics of major depressive disorder. *Current Psychiatry Reports, 2*, 165–169.
7. Caspi, A., Sugden, K., Moffitt, T. E., et al. (2003). Influence of life stress on depression: Moderation by a polymorphism in the 5-HTT gene. *Science, 301*, 386–389.
8. Kendler, K. S., Kuhn, J. W., Vittum, J., et al. (2005). The interaction of stressful life events and a serotonin transporter polymorphism in the prediction of episodes of major depression: A replication. *Archives of General Psychiatry, 62*, 529–535.

9. Gillespie, N. A., Whitfield, J. B., Williams, B., et al. (2005). The relationship between stressful life events, the serotonin transporter (5-HTTLPR) genotype and major depression. *Psychological Medicine, 35*, 101–111.
10. Stokes, P. E. (1993). Fluoxetine: A five-year review. *Clinical Therapeutics, 15*, 216–243.
11. Cole, J. O. (1992). New directions in antidepressant therapy: A review of sertraline, a unique serotonin reuptake inhibitor. *Journal of Clinical Psychiatry, 53*, 333–340.
12. Yuhua, H., Hui, X., Xiaoyan, N., et al. (2024). Association between duration of antidepressant treatment for major depressive disorder and relapse rate after discontinuation: A meta-analysis. *Psychiatry Research, 337*. https://doi.org/10.1016/j.psychres.2024.115926
13. Rice, P. L. (1987). *Stress and health: Principles and practice for coping and wellness*. Brooks/Cole Publishing.
14. Charlesworth, E. A., & Nathan, R. G. (1984). *Stress management: A comprehensive guide to wellness*. Ballantine Books.
15. Koh, K. B. (1999). *Ways to keep myself from all kinds of stressors*. Haneon.
16. Qureshi, F., Soo, J., Chen, Y., et al. (2022). Optimism and lipid profiles in mid-life: A 15-year study of black and white adults. *American Journal of Preventive Medicine, 62*, e169–e177. https://doi.org/10.1016/j-amepre.2021.09.011
17. Boehm, J. K., Williams, D. R., Rimm, E. B., et al. (2013). Relation between optimism and lipids in mid-life. *American Journal of Cardiology, 111*, 1425–1431.
18. Rasmussen, H. N., Scheier, M. F., Greenhouse, J. B., et al. (2009). Optimism and physical health: A meta-analytic review. *Annals of Behavioral Medicine, 37*, 239–256.
19. Whitfield, J. B., Zhu, G., Landers, J. G., et al. (2020). Pessimism is associated with greater all-cause and cardiovascular mortality, but optimism is not protective. *Science and Reports, 10*, 12609. https://doi.org/10.1038/s41598-020-69388-y
20. Frankl, V. E. (2006). *Man's search for meaning*. Beacon Press.
21. WHO. (1992). *Basic documents* (39th ed.). WHO.
22. Ellison, C. G., & Levin, J. S. (1998). The religion-health connection: Evidence, theory, and future directions. *Health Education & Behavior, 25*, 700–720.
23. Mueller, P. S., Plevak, D. J., & Rummans, T. A. (2001). Religious involvement, spirituality, and medicine: Implications for clinical practice. *Mayo Clinic Proceedings, 76*, 1225–1235.
24. Matthews, D. A., McCullough, M. E., Larson, D. B., et al. (1998). Religious commitment and health status: A review of the research and implications for family medicine. *Archives of Family Medicine, 7*, 118–124.

Chapter 3
How to Manage Stress

3.1 The Goals and Principles of Stress Management [1]

The goals of stress management can be divided into three stages: Stage 1 is treatment of illness, Stage 2 is prevention of illness, and Stage 3 is promotion of health and enhancement of quality of life.

The basic principles of stress management are as follows: first, minimize the frequency of stress response; second, minimize the intensity of stress response, and third, use stress.

Social and personality engineering is used to minimize the frequency of stress responses, whereas relaxation training, meditation, and biofeedback are used to minimize the intensity of stress responses. Finally, physical exercise is a way of using stress.

3.1.1 Social Engineering

Social engineering refers to the willful alteration of lifestyle and/or the general environment to minimize exposure to stressors. The primary goal of social engineering is not to change the nature of stressors. For example, if your job is stressful because your boss is overly demanding, it is likely useless to attempt to change the boss. In this example, you can change the amount of time you spend with your boss, change bosses via a transfer, or even consider changing jobs.

Social engineering involves seeking alternatives or modifying one's position in relation to stressors.

For adaptive stress, one can establish routines, use time-blocking techniques, or establish a "mental health" day. When possible, avoid or minimize other changes during periods of massive changes.

For frustration-related stress, find new alternatives to your frustrated goal.

K. B. Koh, *Body, Mind and Spirituality*, https://doi.org/10.1007/978-3-032-11214-9_3

For overload, set priorities, delegate responsibility, enlist the support of others, accept fallibility, determine optimal stress levels, and avoid exposure to stressors.

The best way to determine the optimal stress level is to recognize the signs of distress (mood, visceral, and musculoskeletal signs).

For deprivational stress (boredom and/or loneliness), plan ahead to avoid potentially stressful situations.

For bioecological stress, monitor biorhythms; use nutritional engineering (e.g., limiting caffeine such as coffee and tea; reducing salt intake, chocolate, colas, refined sugar, and processed flour [junk food]); stay away from smoking areas; and avoid exposure to noise.

3.1.2 Personality Engineering

Personality engineering aims to reduce stress by intentionally altering personality traits (behaviors) such as poor self-esteem and depression, anxious reactive personality, and Type A personality.

For those with poor self-esteem and depression, positive verbalization and assertiveness training should be practiced to enhance self-esteem. Positive verbalization refers to the process in which one reinforces one's self-image by pointing out positive aspects of oneself. Assertiveness training can improve self-esteem. Assertiveness is the positive and productive expression of oneself.

Maintaining eye contact is often one of the most difficult tasks for an unassertive person. One may find it awkward at first. The best way to maintain eye contact is to start with short intervals (2–3s in length).

For anxious reactive personalities, one can engage in thought stopping. This technique enables a stressed person to intentionally break the anxiety cycle by abruptly leaving obsessional thoughts. For example, this technique involves shouting the word "Stop!" Another form of thought stopping is to switch abruptly to a pleasing, relaxing image or scene in your mind as soon as you become aware of an anxious cycle.

For those with Type A personality, which is characterized by time urgency, competitiveness, and aggression/hostility, using time management for time urgency helps.

3.1.3 Physical Exercise

It is desirable to exercise without awareness of competition because competition itself can substantially add to the arousal level of exercise. For example, exercises such as walking, running, biking, swimming, and skiing often have greater relaxation rewards than competitive sports, in which winning is more important than playing your best.

3.1.4 Two Rules for Stress Management [2]

Rule No. 1: Do not sweat the small stuff.
Rule No. 2: "It is all small stuff. If you can neither fight nor flee, flow."

3.2 Daily Routine of Muscle Relaxation and Stretching [2]

Relaxation methods can be used to manage anxiety and other stressors. Brief relaxation practices throughout the day can help break the dangerous stress signals. These practice periods may take less than five minutes; however, they can bring great benefits by helping you keep tension below critical levels.

Many people who work in offices experience muscle tension, resulting in headaches, backaches, and shoulder pain. Relaxation helps them release tension and prevent pain.

First, it is recommended to relax the shoulders and neck, which are parts of the body that are likely to be susceptible to muscular tension but difficult to keep relaxed.

1. Interlock your fingers, stretch them forward, take a deep breath, and count one to five.
2. Hold your breath and return to your original position, counting one to five.
3. Unclasp your hands, put them down, slowly breathe out, and count one to five.

As mentioned above, stretch your interlocked fingers backward, take a deep breath, count one to five, and then hold your breath. Bring your fingers back to their original position, counting one to five. Then unclasp your hands, put them down, slowly breathe out, and count one to five.

Likewise, raise your interlocked fingers and stretch them upward and over your head, take a deep breath, and count one to five. Hold your breath and bring your interlocked fingers down to your head, count one to five. Then unclasp your hands, put them down on the surface, slowly breathe out, and count one to five.

Shrug your shoulders up, take a deep breath, and count one to five. Hold your breath in the same posture, count one to five, and then return to your original position. Slowly breathe out and count one to five.

In addition, bend your neck backward, take a deep breath, count one to five, and then hold your breath in the same posture. Count one to five. Return to your original position, slowly breathe out, and count one to five.

Whenever you breathe out, say, "Relax" or "let go." It is also good to recall or imagine beautiful scenery.

Perform stretching and muscle relaxation for five minutes, if possible, whenever you finish working for an hour. This helps relax muscular tension and enhance work efficiency.

Practice stretching and muscle relaxation at least three times a day, even when you do not work. This helps effectively relieve the tension of the body and mind.

3.3 Physical and Psychological Effects of Exercise

Regular exercise is not only good for physical health but also for psychological health.

3.3.1 Physical Benefits of Exercise [3, 4]

Regular exercise lowers blood pressure by reducing peripheral resistance, decreases low-density lipoprotein and serum cholesterol levels, reduces the risk of heart attacks, and improves the functioning of the circulatory system. It also increases respiratory capacity and muscle tone, improves immune functions [2], and slows the aging process [5].

These effects can increase endurance and lower fatigue [3]. In addition, exercise is effective in the prevention of dementia, as well as in the treatment and prevention of adult diseases such as diabetes, hypertension, heart disease, and osteoporosis [6].

3.3.2 Psychological Benefits of Exercise

Exercise has positive psychological effects. Exercise can enhance self-esteem by reducing body weight and improving body image. It also improves sleep and mental functioning (e.g., concentration and efficiency) and induces relief from mild depression [7] and anxiety [8].

Exercise can help you manage stress by reducing the secretion of noradrenaline caused by stressors, resulting in decreased stress-related behaviors [9]. Endorphins are released in great abundance by the brain during exercise, such as jogging or long-distance running, leading to euphoria and relaxation of muscles [3].

Exercise can also enhance creativity. In particular, exercise is effective in diverting attention from work overload or difficult and stressful situations.

3.3.3 Start with Exercises You Can Easily Do

If you are not ready to do a specific exercise and have no time to do it, you can start with exercises you can easily do. For example, you can take the stairs instead of elevators or make a detour rather than take a short cut. Additionally, muscle-strengthening exercises such as weightlifting (using dumbbells), push-ups, and squats should be performed to reduce the risk of osteoporosis and strengthen muscles [10, 11].

Walking at least three times a week for more than 40 min each time or twice for 20 min is recommended. In terms of the effect of exercise, it is desirable to feel a slight increase in the heartbeat when walking. If you cannot exercise outside, you can walk taking long strides in your office or room.

3.4 Listen to Your Body Signals: Thirst Cues

Drinking enough water is crucial for overall health. Healthy adults require approximately 35 ml of water per kg of body weight per day [12]. An individual weighing 50 kg requires 1.7 L; 60 kg, 2.1 L; 70 kg, 2.4 L; and 80 kg, 2.8 L. This includes fluids from plain water, beverages such as teas and juice, and food. An average of 20 percent of one's water intake occurs from food sources [13]. Therefore, a person weighing 60 kg needs to drink approximately 1.7 L (7 cups of a 250 ml cup) of water a day after excluding fluid from food (2,100 ml minus 420 ml). However, the amount of water required also depends on an individual's level of activity (e.g., exercise) and climate (hot weather) [14, 15].

Drinking a cup of water immediately after waking is recommended because it helps prevent dehydration by replenishing the fluids lost from the body (through urine, respiration, and perspiration) after a night of sleep. Water plays a vital role in maintaining healthy skin, digestion, and body temperature [14, 15]. In addition, it helps eliminate waste through urine, sweat, and bowel movements [16], lose body weight [17], maintain blood pressure [17, 18], and improve cognitive function [19].

Dehydration, caused by insufficient water intake, can lead to various health issues, including fatigue, constipation, and even more serious conditions like kidney stones (e.g., colicky abdominal pain) or urinary tract infections (e.g., back pain) [20, 21]. Therefore, it is important to pay attention to thirst cues (e.g., dry mouth, dark yellow urine, decreased urination, dizziness, and fatigue) and drink water with and between meals throughout the day to maintain hydration.

However, excessive water intake should be avoided, as it can lead to dangerous conditions such as hyponatremia (low sodium levels in the blood), which may cause symptoms such as nausea, headaches, confusion, seizures, and even death due to cerebral edema [22]. Compulsive water drinking has been linked to a broad spectrum of psychopathologies, ranging from mild neurosis to psychosis (e.g., chronic schizophrenic disorder) [23]. Mental health professionals should, therefore, pay attention to and evaluate the water intake behaviors of chronic inpatients.

3.5 How to Avoid Overeating: Mindful Eating

Overeating can cause stomach pain and indigestion, alter the regulation of hunger, and contribute to weight gain. Being overweight is a significant health risk factor for obesity, heart disease, and type 2 diabetes [24].

Eating has often become a mindless act performed quickly. This can be problematic because it takes time (about 20 min) for the brain to register that you are full.

Leptin is a hormone that acts as the body's satiety signal and works in opposition to ghrelin, another hormone that stimulates appetite. Together, these hormones help regulate energy balance and food intake [25].

If one eats too fast, the fullness signal may not arrive until they have already consumed too much food. This is common among people who overeat. Distractions (e.g., watching television and using smartphones) may also contribute to excessive eating [26, 27].

By eating mindfully, the individual pays close attention to their body's hunger and fullness cues while eating and slows their eating, making it an intentional act rather than an automatic one. Mindful eating helps an individual differentiate between true hunger and emotional or external cues to eat. Sensory eating reduces food intake by slowing one's eating rate [28]. In addition, utilizing external cues (e.g., reducing portion sizes and distractions while eating) helps achieve awareness [29]. This intervention helps one lose weight by changing their eating behaviors and reducing stress [30–32].

Mindful eating can improve digestion by encouraging one to chew food thoroughly and pay attention to the eating process (e.g., the taste, texture, and smell of food) and the overall eating experience. This can lead to more satisfactory and complete meals. Therefore, mindful eating is an effective intervention for weight control [33–35].

3.6 How to Deal with Anger

Anger is an emotion people most frequently experience. The manner in which anger is managed differs from person to person. Some people drink alcohol, smoke cigarettes, or scold their children, while others harm themselves or assault others.

However, some people suppress their anger, resulting in somatic symptoms such as aching all over and visiting clinics or hospitals.

3.6.1 Anger Is Poison; You Get Ill If You Suppress Anger

People who tend to hold their anger are more prone to illnesses such as cancer, irritable bowel syndrome, hypertension, and tension headaches. *Hwa-byung* is known as an anger syndrome specific to Korean culture, which is attributed to anger suppression and is characterized by various somatic symptoms, including a feeling of a mass in the epigastrium and hot sensation [36].

Hostile individuals are at high risk of developing coronary heart disease [37]. Compared to healthy individuals, patients with hypertension are more likely to experience anger suppression rather than anger expression [38]. You cannot maintain your health by suppressing your anger. This is because anger is revealed somewhere in the body when it is not verbally expressed.

Case 1

A 50-year-old woman continuously suffered from lower abdominal pain and diarrhea. She therefore visited the department of internal medicine of a university hospital, where no laboratory abnormalities were found. She was referred to the department of psychiatry for consultation. Thereafter, she was several times admitted to psychiatry via the emergency room because of repetitive abdominal pain and diarrhea. According to her family, her husband had an extramarital affair with another woman who gave birth to a son. Then the patient took care of the son for a period of 20 years while her husband was living with the woman. Recently her husband got back home. At that time, she began to develop her symptoms.

This suggests that her large bowel symptoms are likely to be associated with her suppressed hostility toward her husband.

Case 2

A man in his early 30s was referred to the department of psychiatry via the department of neurology, where he complained of severe headache. Later he said, "my superior used to scold me whenever outcomes were not perfect." Moreover, the head interfered in a lot of trivial things. He felt afraid of reporting to the superior. He couldn't say anything to the superior.

It is desirable to hold back anger to some degree; however, suppressing anger too much can make you ill. Therefore, one needs to find a way to properly release anger.

3.6.2 Anger Is Addictive

If anger is so often expressed, it becomes a habit. In the end, anger begets anger. Living with a hostile person can lead to hostility, as it is highly infectious.

For example, a man in his 30s was physically abused by his father. Later, after his marriage, he beats his wife for trivial reasons.

Moreover, venting anger on someone wrongly is the worst way to deal with anger.

A woman in her 20s became angry with her mother-in-law, who said, "Why did you get married if you would like to go out to meet your friends? You have many things to do at home." She was not permitted to get a job. She often breaks things and beats her child. She then felt remorse about her faults and cried.

After all, shooting a messenger increases stress, provoking anger, and creating a vicious cycle.

3.6.3 What Makes Us Hostile?

Researchers have found that individuals with a history of aggressive behavior have reduced levels of the major breakdown product of serotonin in their brain and spinal cord, suggesting an association between low serotonin function and aggressive behavior [39].

In animal studies, low serotonin function is expected to increase sympathetic nervous system activity and decrease parasympathetic nervous system activity. A similar pattern was observed in hostile persons [39].

Anger has long been associated with depression. Patients with depressive disorders have been reported to experience more anger attacks than healthy volunteers [40]. Patients with depressive disorders were also found to be more likely to experience anger than those with anxiety or somatic symptom and related disorders [41].

3.6.4 A Strategy to Reduce Anger [39]

The following are two rules to live by to reduce anger:

1. Do not sweat the small suff.
2. Most matters are small stuff.

Many hostile people begin with inappropriate thoughts about others or situations that cannot be changed. By learning to reason with yourself, you can often talk to yourself out of cynical thoughts, angry feelings, and aggressive behaviors. This skill is used as the starting point for all subsequent strategies.

3.6.5 Have an Internal Dialogue [39]

Many people do not know how to manage anger, as they often experience it. When you feel angry, talk to yourself.

First, ask yourself, "If I am angry about something, is the matter worth my continued attention?".

Most of the matter is small. For example, if a beggar talks abusively to you on the street, it will make you angry; however, it is not as important as it is worth your continued attention. In this case, you can pass by the beggar saying, "That guy is strange!".

Next, ask yourself, "Am I justified?" If a colleague continues to insult you every day, you will become upset and angry. This situation is not only worth your continued attention but your anger can also be justified.

Then ask, "Do I have an effective response?" If one is confident in doing so, one can assert oneself.

However, self-assertion should be considered as a last resort after trying other things: (a) thought stopping, distraction, and meditation/relaxation as ways to deflect anger; (b) empathy, tolerance, and forgiveness as ways to improve relationships; and (c) humor, religion, and "pretend today is your last" as ways to adopt positive attitude.

If you are convinced that you can change your colleague's attitude, doing so will be effective. However, if he is your boss, it will be better to change your own view or attitude rather than make an assertion.

Ignore minor things; however, if you are too angry to tolerate, go to the person who arouses your ire and express your thoughts or feelings.

Case 1

A woman in her early 40s was submissive to her husband and endured his nagging since marriage. Recently, however, she even thought of divorce and started to say what she wanted to say and cried out, "I will leave you if you continue to interfere in trivial things." Thereafter, the woman felt better, and her husband stopped nagging her.

Case 2

Another woman in her 40s had endured her husband's unreasonable and unconditional demand, but for the first time, she defied him and was then slapped on the face. What was strange was that she felt relieved rather than bad.

As such, it is the last bastion of your mental health to express your feelings rather than suppress them, even if it may annoy your husband.

If you are angry, have an internal dialogue on the following: (1) whether the matter is important, (2) whether you are justified, and (3) whether you have an effective response.

If you say, "No," you need to reason with yourself. Nevertheless, if you continue to be angry, try to stop thinking, distract yourself, meditate, and relax.

Thereafter, try to have empathy, tolerance, and forgiveness. In addition, humor, prayers, and "pretend today is your last" may help relieve anger.

3.7 How to Foster Positive Thinking

3.7.1 A Failure at Work Is not a Failure of Life [6]

Long ago, a first-year medical student who had done well in premedical course committed suicide by jumping through the window of the room at a hotel where he was staying. Around the same time, the vice president of a large company took his life by jumping from the roof of a high-rise apartment. In addition to work overload, he was frustrated after being transferred from research director to plant manager. Another female high school student jumped to her death from an apartment after finding that her test scores were low. The key problem in all these cases was that they regarded their failure at work as a failure of life.

People sometimes anticipate failure at work and feel anxious. A newspaper reported that a female college student who entered university at the top of her class and maintained first place during her freshman year committed suicide. Presumably, this was because she was afraid of losing the first place. The goal of her life was to obtain first place. It was assumed that she did not find pleasure in things other than getting the first place.

Why do people who do well at school, attend a good university, or work at a good company commit suicide? This is probably because such suicides may be associated with impaired emotion regulation and decision-making, as well as impaired cognitive control owing to structural and functional deficits in the prefrontal cortex [42–47].

Moreover, such individuals who do well are unlikely to seek help from others. In particular, as a last resort, they are vulnerable to suicide because they usually have no social support system that offers comfort and advice (e.g., family members or friends).

Behind most successful people are numerous failures. For example, accepting initial failures or setbacks as part of the trial-and-error process will bring one closer to becoming a successful stress manager [2].

3.7.2 Check Your Life Goals [6]

Work can be a way to make life abundant, but it cannot be your life goal. Success in work can give you temporary pleasure but does not guarantee your happiness continually. If work itself is the goal of life, the price will be self-destructive.

Overall, we learn and grow through trial and error. We enhance our immunity against failures through the experience of falling and standing. The failures and trials of an individual or a nation may become opportunities to mature.

Life is always by no means smooth sailing. At first, everything is done well, but you may get frustrated in the middle; while you may not do well at first, you may do well at the last.

In a competitive society, where only people getting first place are remembered, many suicidal cases teach us to live by setting a bigger goal in life and trying hard to achieve in an individual's work. We need to have the habit of looking back on the past to check whether we are moving toward our goal in life.

Individually, one can feel a sense of achievement anywhere other than work or school. One can obtain satisfaction through hobbies, exercise, friends, and group or religious activities. Thus, having an interest in things other than work can make life happy and abundant.

3.7.3 Change Your Thinking Habit [6]

Often, what we inadvertently say or show tends to be out of habit. This is because our thinking has a certain rule or framework, regardless of whether it is conscious or unconscious.

Automatically responding according to the rules or frameworks of our thoughts, we say the same words or behave repetitively in response to the same stimulus. This thinking habit can bring some people success but others failure.

An employee in his 30s was often helpless, saying, "I am incompetent" without checking whether he is right whenever he was blamed by his superior.

He would say, "I am incompetent" when his subordinates did not follow what he said. He would also blame himself and would say so, even when his team lost in the inter-division football game. He automatically says the same thing whenever he encounters an unpleasant event.

Another case is a professor who often says, "That is my fault," regardless of personal or departmental problems.

He was agonized by feeling inadequate as a professor and carried many books home whenever he left work. Someone close to him called him the "Living Jesus."

When one lives overburdened, it causes serious harm to the body, particularly to the heart. He died of myocardial infarction in his early 50s.

Our thinking habits dominate our words and behaviors and affect our health. Therefore, it is not an exaggeration to say that thinking becomes the seed for our words and behaviors and finally determines our destiny.

First, observe what words you inadvertently and repetitively say and then check whether they harm your health and distress others. If so, try to change your words consciously.

3.7.4 Effects of Laughter

Laughter is an elixir that maintains health. Laughter relieves tension and anxiety, improves blood circulation, releases endorphins known as natural pain relievers, enhances immune function, and prevents diseases [48]. People who live a long time do not lose their smile.

In contrast, those who are pessimistic and depressed are likely to develop diseases because their immune functions are reduced [49–52]. In particular, those who neither laugh nor express their emotions are at risk of cancer [53–56].

A woman in her early 50s was distressed because her husband cheated on her several times. Not long ago, she had suffered from headaches and did not have much to live when such events came to mind.

However, she changed her mind and decided to live with smiles after saying to herself, "How long can I live?" Thereafter, she was pleasant and smiling continuously.

Sometimes, she would visit a neighbor with cancer and took care of the patient. However, this was not difficult for her.

Making a conscious effort to explore humorous things and exposure to fun events help enhance resilience. Additionally, it is a good way to recall someone who appears to be fun. For example, one comedian said, "I am sorry to have bad looks," making him famous as a great comedian.

3.7.5 How to Nurture a Positive Language Habit

Optimists are not only more likely to succeed in society than pessimists but are also known to suffer from depression or physical diseases less than pessimists [6].

The importance of optimistic thinking is to prevent people from becoming lost in negative thinking and helpless and to give them the strength to overcome difficulties.

Learned helplessness often leads to depression among pessimists who have experienced failure. However, failure can only temporarily let optimists down.

Seligman [57] believed that individuals have their own language habits. In other words, when something bad occurs, individuals use their own language to explain it.

According to these language habits, some individuals are optimistic, whereas others are pessimistic. A pessimistic explanatory style diffuses helplessness, whereas an optimistic explanatory style interrupts it. Therefore, helplessness depends on how mistakes or frustrations faced in daily life are explained.

Pessimists' language habit means that explanation for something bad is personal ("That is my fault"), permanent ("This always happens"), and pervasive ("This will mess up everything in my life").

If you talk about your failures continuously and pervasively, you are likely to make mistakes in the future again. For example, a man rejected by a woman he loved would say, "Women dislike me" (pervasive) and "I will not meet women" (permanent). The problem with these two factors related to the language habits of pessimists is that a man thinks he will be rejected continuously, not only by his lover but also by every woman.

Therefore, pessimists who want to become optimists must change their language habits. In other words, the best way for pessimists to become optimists is to change their destructive thinking or language habits whenever they experience frustration [57].

For example, when pessimists are not promoted, they respond, "I am finished. I will not be at work anymore. I am not confident in getting along with my family." By contrast, optimists do not allow frustration to influence their life. They usually respond, "I am in low spirit because I am not promoted. I will work harder and then I will look for another job if I am not promoted again."

3.7.6 *Play to Your Strengths*

We tend to spend a lot of time looking for the worst in ourselves and correcting them. This is because we have the wrong belief that we should correct our weaknesses instead of playing to our strengths. However, you will not only spend your life correcting your bad habits, but it is also not easy to root it out [6].

Occasionally, an individual's strength can be a weakness, or vice versa. Some regard stubbornness as a weakness but consider tenacity and perseverance as strengths. Stubbornness or tenacity can become either a weakness or strength, depending on which word is chosen. In other words, tenacity can be viewed as painting stubbornness in a good light. The secret to rapid success is to play to your strength (tenacity) rather than clinging to your weakness (stubbornness) [6].

In a long-term prospective study of people with high intelligence quotient (IQ: an average IQ of 150), psychologists found that intellect and achievement were far from perfectly correlated and that personality traits such as perseverance and goal-directed behavior were more prominent in the most successful people than in the least successful ones [58, 59]. Based on evaluation of educational attainment by adults, Duckworth et al. [60] reported that grit, defined as "perseverance and passion for long-term goals," as a personality trait, is a better predictor of success than intellectual talent (IQ).

In other words, those who were remarkably successful devoted themselves to what they wanted to do. They were those who made the most of their strengths.

3.7.7 *How to Overcome Anthropophobia (Fear of People) [6]*

Some people feel an intense fear or anxiety about being around others. Their faces appear rigid, and their hands and feet tremble. They also had difficulty making eye contact, avoiding other people.

Most of them usually have painful experiences, such as injury to their self-esteem in interpersonal relationships or in front of many people.

A woman in her mid-40s was afraid of making eye contact and felt uncomfortable when meeting people face-to-face.

She was unable to visit the bank because she felt uncomfortable with others. One day, she was supposed to meet her son's high school teacher. At the time, she felt anxious because she did not know what to say. She also felt smaller when meeting her friend who was smarter and richer than her. She became depressed and felt chest discomfort even when her friends talked about their children, who were superior to her son.

She had been pent-up for a long time, as she had been treated, unlike her older sister during childhood. Her mother would push her hands away while embracing and hugging her sister. During elementary school, her mother would visit her sister's class but not her class. Moreover, her side dish was different from that of her sister.

Such painful experiences, in which she had been rejected by her mother in the past, came back to haunt her. The scar had remained in her heart for a long time, even after her son entered college. Therefore, she could not like her mother.

Past experiences, such as being rejected, continue to be brought back like nightmares, causing fear of people and avoidance. Moreover, when individuals are overwhelmed by numerous demands—particularly those involving interpersonal relationships—they may become more vulnerable to developing such a phobia.

Strenuous efforts of singers, dancers, and famous emcees are not seen on stage. Fear of people can be managed by practicing interpersonal relationship skills, along with gradual exposure to people.

Consider what you need to say when meeting people, write a memo in advance, memorize it, and practice it like an actor. This will help you gain confidence and overcome fear of people by reducing your scars.

3.8 Workaholism

3.8.1 Recognize Signs of Burnout

Excessive work and frequent frustration can lead to physical and emotional exhaustion. This syndrome is known as burnout. Burnout appears to be a major factor in low worker morale, high absenteeism and job turnover rates, physical illness and distress, increased alcohol and drug use, marital and family conflicts, and various psychological problems [3].

Symptoms of burnout include increased physical complaints, social withdrawal, emotional exhaustion, loss of self-esteem, depression, frustration, and feeling trapped. Burnout may be characterized by pessimism, paranoia, rigidity, callousness, feelings of loneliness and guilt, and difficulties in making and explaining decisions [61–63].

Case

A man in his early 40s was supposed to be named department head but felt stifled, alienated, and frustrated because he was excluded from meetings where important decisions related to his department were made. He would get easily annoyed over many trivial things in his department. He said, “I would like to live a brainless life.” He did not want to exercise or take trips he used to enjoy. He even thought about going to another company if it allowed him to do his job.

The signs and symptoms of burnout are warning signals of overstress. In such cases, you need to take steps to improve your health and safety before doing other things as soon as possible. First, move away from job commitment. Then consult a mental health professional. Simultaneously, focus on managing stress by taking rest, relaxation, meditation, vacations, or trips.

3.8.2 *Get Enough Rest [48]*

God created the heaven and earth in six days and then rested. Therefore, it is natural and necessary to rest once a week. Without rest, we cannot maintain health or survive. Rest helps increase productivity and enhances creativity.

Sometimes, entering the mountains is not permitted as they require rest. Even rocks are occasionally protected by banning access to them.

Some people suffer from illnesses without resting when they need to. Moreover, among those who only worked hard without rest in the past, quite a few people often made a great fortune but lost their health.

If you work too much on weekdays, it is good to get enough rest for one day during the weekend. If you suffer from a lack of sleep on weekdays, get enough sleep on weekends.

Rest is vital to maintain general good health and handle stress. However, it is often challenging to get enough rest when stressed because stressful situations (e.g., work and personal concerns) may disturb the ability to rest. In this case, you must have the courage to make choices that help you get enough rest, even if this is a challenge.

Here are some tips to help you rest effectively.

Rest from Your Work

Plan to give yourself at least one day each week when you do not do any work; give yourself time outside of your work responsibilities. If staying home means you will have to work, plan an outing far away from work opportunities.

Rest by Sleeping

Sleep not only provides rest but also allows the brain to replenish essential biochemicals (e.g., growth hormone and melatonin), which help us cope with stress. The increased secretion of growth hormone during deep (slow-wave) sleep is essential for tissue repair and regeneration [64, 65]. An increase in melatonin levels at night promotes sleepiness and regulates the sleep-wake cycle [66–68].

Adequate sleep is important for both physical (cardiovascular, cerebrovascular, and metabolic health) and mental well-being. It also leads to improved mood, better concentration, enhanced cognitive function (e.g., memory and decision-making), and a reduced risk of accidents and injuries [69–71]. Therefore, sleep is closely associated with emotional resilience.

Although stress can cause sleep difficulties, take the following steps to ensure that you get enough rest:

1. Establish a regular sleep-wake schedule.
2. Do not drink anything containing caffeine four hours before bedtime.
3. Avoid alcohol and nicotine before bedtime.

Many people tend to drink alcohol to induce sleep, but this actually disrupts it. Initially, it may help alcohol users fall asleep faster, but later impairs both the quality and quantity of sleep, particularly in regular alcohol users. Alcohol interferes with the natural sleep cycle, particularly by reducing rapid eye movement (REM) sleep, which is crucial for memory consolidation and emotional regulation. This can result in more frequent awakenings throughout the night [72–76].

4. Limit water intake at least two hours before bedtime [77].

Limiting water intake before bedtime helps reduce the need to urinate at night, thereby minimizing sleep disruptions.

5. Set electronic devices aside at least an hour before bedtime.

Phones, computers, TVs, and other electronic devices with screens emit blue light, which can disrupt the body's production of melatonin and make it difficult to fall asleep [78].

6. Reduce vigorous physical or mental activity before bed. Instead, do stretching and relaxation.
7. If you have trouble falling asleep, get up and do relaxation by listening to soothing music.

Rest Periodically

Schedule periods of regular rest. While working for an hour in a day, do a relaxing activity you enjoy for five minutes. Take time for your own rest one day in a week.

Take a Break from Environment Creating Tensions

If a particular place is too tense, take a break by removing yourself from the place until you are able to regain your composure.

Rest from Excessive External Stimuli

Set aside a period of time when you cut out all the noise, turn off the television, and leave your mobile phone. When you relieve yourself of all external stimuli, you will be better able to listen to what is going on inside you—that is, your inner needs.

3.8.3 Work 70%–80% of Your Maximum Capacity to Do

Workaholics enjoy work and therefore may not notice the harm it is doing (e.g., on their relationships or health). Excessive work, even if enjoyed, can be an occupational stressor. Workaholics tend to be energetic, sleep less than most people, have difficulty taking rest or vacations, spend most of their waking time working, prefer working to playing, tend to blur the distinction between work and play, and work anytime and anywhere [3]

They place more value on work than on any other thing. They get mad at work, saying, "If I have no work, what makes me live?" Workaholics do not get away from work, similar to alcoholics or drug addicts who do not get away from drinking alcohol or taking drugs.

They may be successful at work but tend to lose many other things. Working hard most of the time not only makes them ache all over but also does not let them know how efficient and productive their work is.

Excessive work is likely to cause marital conflict. Workaholics do not spend time with their family members; therefore, they tend to feel left alone.

They also do not know how stressed they are when they are engaged in work, resulting in harm to their health. These individuals are known to be at high risk of coronary heart disease. To prevent workaholism, it is desirable to work at 70%–80% of maximum capacity. Schedule to limit activities to a few things per day. If there are things they have not done that day, it is better to skip those things and do them the next day.

3.9 Enjoy Loneliness; Otherwise, Get Away from It [6]

Creative people enjoy loneliness. Loneliness gives one the opportunity to look into oneself and grow mentally. Moreover, people who believe in God may develop close relationships with him by praying, which helps them grow spiritually.

If you like to be lonely, do not intentionally try to get along with others. Such compulsive acts may hurt you.

However, an individual who is intolerant of being alone, and hence likes to talk to anyone, is vulnerable to anxiety or depression on facing loneliness. Bereaved husbands and wives are likely to develop diseases or die earlier because their immune functions are weakened by loneliness [79–82].

Case 1

A woman in her late 60s was admitted to the internal medicine department of a hospital and was referred to the department of psychiatry. She had been treated for a duodenal ulcer at the internal medicine department for approximately 20 years. However, recently, her symptoms were aggravated. The reason for referral was to determine whether the aggravation was psychologically related.

After an interview, she was found to suffer more severe symptoms when she began to feel lonely after her tenant, who used to talk with her, got a job and went out, leaving her alone.

Case 2
A woman in her early 40s visited the emergency room (ER) several times a month complaining of anxiety while her husband was working in a Middle Eastern country. Every time she visited the ER, she experienced dizziness, chest tightness, difficulty in breathing, and extreme fear along with a sense of impending death. She was referred to the department of psychiatry and was diagnosed with panic disorder.

Thereafter, she never visited the hospital for approximately a month. Later, however, she visited the department of psychiatry again and said, "I did not have such symptoms anymore while my husband was back home." However, her symptoms recurred after her husband left the home country.

As seen in this case, feelings of loneliness can be perceived as death. If people want to stay healthy and live longer, they need to get along with others. The following are some tips for you:

Eat lunch with others. Otherwise, you can telephone them, write letters, and promote friendships through hobby club activities and study or religious groups. Occasionally, volunteer work can also help avoid loneliness.

3.10 Summary

1. The goals of stress management can be divided into three stages: Stage 1 is treatment of illness, Stage 2 is prevention of illness, and Stage 3 is promotion of health and enhancement of quality of life.
2. The basic principles of stress management are as follows: first, minimize the frequency of stress response; second, minimize the intensity of stress response; and finally, use stress.
3. Along with daily routines of muscle relaxation and stretching, physical and psychological effects of exercise were reviewed.
4. How to manage anger, workaholism, and loneliness and foster positive thinking were mainly addressed in this chapter.

References

1. Girdano, D. A., & Everly, G. (1979). *Controlling stress and tension: A holistic approach.* Prentice-Hall.
2. Charlesworth, E. A., & Nathan, R. G. (1984). *Stress management: A comprehensive guide to wellness.* Ballantine Books.
3. Greenberg, J. S. (1990). *Coping with stress: A practical guide.* Wm. C. Brown Publishers.
4. Rice, P. L. (1987). *Stress and health: Principles and practice for coping and wellness.* Brooks/Cole Publishing.
5. Harris, R., Frankel, L. J., & Harris, S. (Eds.). (1977). *Guide to fitness after fifty.* Plenum Press.
6. Koh, K. B. (1999). *Ways to keep myself from all kinds of stressors.* Haneon.

7. Corbin, C. B., & Lindsey, R. (1988). *Concepts of physical fitness with laboratories* (6th ed.). Wm. C. Brown Publishers.
8. Mikevic, P. (1982). Anxiety, depression and exercise. *Quest, 33*, 140–153.
9. Stone, W. J. (1987). *Adult fitness programs: Planning, designing, managing, and improving fitness programs*. Scott, Foresman and Company.
10. Beck, B. R., Daly, R. M., Singh, M. A. F., et al. (2017). Exercise and Sports Science Australia (ESSA) position statement on exercise prescription for the prevention and management of osteoporosis. *Journal of Science and Medicine in Sport, 20*, 438–445.
11. Kohrt, W. M., Bloomfield, S. A., Little, K. D., et al. (2004). Physical activity and bone health. *Medicine & Science in Sports & Exercise, 36*, 1985–1996.
12. Mallett, L. J., Premkumar, V., Brown, L. J., et al. (2021). Total water intake by kilogram of body weight: Analysis of the Australian 2011 to 2013 national nutrition and physical activity survey. *Journal of the Dietitians Australia, 78*, 496–505.
13. National Academies of Sciences, Engineering, and Medicine. (2005). *Dietary reference intakes for water, potassium, sodium, chloride, and sulfate*. The National Academies Press.
14. Nakamura, Y., Watanabe, H., Tanaka, A., et al. (2020). Effect of increased daily water intake and hydration. *Nutrients, 12*, 1–17.
15. Sawka, M. N., Cheuvront, S. N., & Carter, R., 3rd. (2005). Human water needs. *Nutrition Reviews, 63*, S30–S39.
16. Jequier, E., & Constant, F. (2010). Water as an essential nutrient: The physiological basis of hydration. *European Journal of Nutrition, 64*, 115–123.
17. Hakam, N., Fuentes, J. L. G., Nabavizadeh, B., et al. (2024). Outcomes in randomized clinical trials testing changes in daily water intake: A systematic review. *JAMA Network Open, 7*(11), e2447621. https://doi.org/10.1001/jamanetworkopen.2024.47621
18. Nakamura, Y., Watanabe, H., Tanaka, A., et al. (2020). Effect of increased daily water intake and hydration on health in Japanese adults. *Nutrients, 12*(4), 1191. https://doi.org/10.3390/nu12041191
19. Benton, D., & Burgess, N. (2009). The effect of the consumption of water on the memory and attention of children. *Appetite, 53*, 143–146.
20. Pearle, M. S., Goldfarb, D. S., Assimos, D. G., et al. (2014). Medical management of kidney stones: AUA guideline. *Journal of Urology, 192*, 316–324.
21. Mitra, P., Pal, D. K., & Das, M. (2018). Does quality of drinking water matter in kidney stone disease: A study in West Bengal, India. *Investigative and Clinical Urology, 59*, 158–165.
22. Sterns, R. H. (2015). Disorders of plasma sodium-causes, consequences, and correction. *New England Journal of Medicine, 372*, 55–65.
23. Singh, S., Padi, M. H., Bullard, H., et al. (1985). Water intoxication in psychiatric patients. *British Journal of Psychiatry, 146*, 127–131.
24. Guh, D. P., Zhang, W., Bansback, N., et al. (2009). The incidence of co-morbidities related to obesity and overweight: A systematic review and meta-analysis. *BMC Public Health, 9*, 88.
25. Zhang, F., Chen, Y., Heiman, M., et al. (2005). Leptin: Structure, function and biology. *Vitamins and Hormones, 71*, 345–372.
26. Ogden, J., Coop, N., Cousins, C., et al. (2013). Distraction, the desire to eat and food intake. Towards an expanded model of mindless eating. *Appetite, 62*, 119–126.
27. Temple, J. L., Giacomelli, A. M., Kent, K. M., et al. (2007). Television watching increases motivated responding for food and energy intake in children. *The American Journal of Clinical Nutrition, 85*, 355–361.
28. Seguias, L., Ferriday, D., Hinton, E. C., et al. (2025). Mindful eating and food intake: Effects and mechanisms of action. *Journal of Experimental Psychology: Applied, 31*, 168–187.
29. Monroe, J. T. (2015). Mindful eating: Principles and practice. *American Journal of Lifestyle Medicine, 9*, 217–220.
30. Dalen, J., Smith, B. W., Shelley, B. M., et al. (2010). Pilot study: Mindful eating and living (MEAL): Weight, eating behavior, and psychological outcomes associated with a mindfulness-based intervention for people with obesity. *Complementary Therapies in Medicine, 18*, 260–264.

31. Timmerman, G. M., & Brown, A. (2012). The effect of a mindful restaurant eating intervention on weight management in women. *Journal of Nutrition Education and Behavior, 44*, 22–28.
32. O'Reilly, G., Cook, L., Spruijt-Metz, D., et al. (2014). Mindfulness-based interventions for obesity-related eating behaviours: A literature review. *Obesity Reviews, 15*, 453–461.
33. Carriere, K., Khoury, B., Gunak, M. M., et al. (2018). Mindfulness-based interventions for weight loss: A systematic review and meta-analysis. *Obesity Reviews, 19*, 164–177.
34. Ruffault, A., Czernichow, S., Hagger, M. S., et al. (2017). The effects of mindfulness training on weight-loss and health-related behaviours in adults with overweight and obesity: A systematic review and meta-analysis. *Obesity Research & Clinical Practice, 11*, 90–111.
35. Katterman, S. N., Kleinman, B. M., Hood, M. M., et al. (2014). Mindfulness meditation as an intervention for binge eating, emotional eating, and weight loss: A systematic review. *Eating Behaviors, 15*, 197–204.
36. Koh, K. B. (2002). *Stress and psychosomatic medicine*. Ilchokak.
37. Hecker, M. H. L., Chesney, M. A., Black, G. W., et al. (1988). Coronary-prone behaviors in the Western Collaborative Group Study. *Psychosomatic Medicine, 50*, 153–164.
38. Koh, K. B., & Kim, S. J. (1995). Comparison of anger between patients with essential hypertension and normal controls. *Korean Journal of Psychosomatic Medicine, 3*, 19–27.
39. Williams, R., & Williams, V. (1993). *Anger kills: Seventeen strategies for controlling the hostility that can harm your health*. Times Books.
40. Fava, M., Rosenbaum, J. F., McCarthy, M., et al. (1991). Anger attacks in depressed outpatients and their response to fluoxetine. *Psychopharmacology Bulletin, 27*, 235–239.
41. Koh, K. B., Kim, C. H., & Park, J. K. (2002). Predominance of anger in depressive disorder compared to anxiety disorder and somatoform disorder. *The Journal of Clinical Psychiatry, 63*, 486–492.
42. Willeumier, K., Taylor, D. V., & Amen, D. G. (2011). Decreased cerebral blood flow in the limbic and prefrontal cortex using SPECT imaging in a cohort of completed suicides. *Translational Psychiatry, 1*, Article e28.
43. Underwood, M. D., Kassir, S. A., Bakalian, M. J., et al. (2012). Neuron density and serotonin receptor binding in prefrontal cortex in suicide. *International Journal of Neuropsychopharmacology, 15*, 435–447.
44. Bludau, S., Eickhoff, S. B., Mohlberg, H., et al. (2014). Cytoarchitecture, probability maps and functions of the human frontal pole. *NeuroImage, 93*, 260–275.
45. Bramson, B., Folloni, D., Verhagen, L., et al. (2020). Human lateral frontal pole contributes to control over emotional approach-avoidance actions. *Journal of Neuroscience, 40*, 2925–2934.
46. van Velzen, L. S., Dauvermann, M. R., Colic, L., et al. (2022). Structural brain alterations associated with suicidal thoughts and behaviors in young people: Results from 21 international studies from the ENIGMA suicidal thoughts and behaviors consortium. *Molecular Psychiatry, 27*, 4550–4560.
47. Gifuni, A. J., Perret, L. C., Lacourse, E., et al. (2020). Decision-making and cognitive control in adolescent suicidal behaviors: A qualitative systematic review of the iterature. *European Child & Adolescent Psychiatry*. https://doi.org/10.1007/s00787-020-01550-3
48. Neal, C. (1993). *52 ways to reduce stress in your life*. Thomas Nelson Publishers.
49. Kronfol, A., Silva, J., Gredin, J., et al. (1983). Impaired lymphocyte function in depressive illness. *Life Sciences, 33*, 241–247.
50. Kronfol, Z., & House, J. D. (1984). Depression, cortisol, and immune function. *Lancet, 1*, 1026–1027.
51. Krueger, R. B., Levy, E. M., & Cathcart, E. S. (1984). Lymphocyte subsets in patients with major depression: Preliminary findings. *Advances, 1*, 5–9.
52. Stein, M., Keller, S. E., & Schleifer, S. J. (1985). Stress and immunomodulation: The role of depression and neuroendocrine function. *Journal of Immunology, 135*, 827–833.
53. Koh, K. B. (1991). A comparison of illness behavior between cancer and noncancer patients. *Journal of Korean Neuropsychiatric Association, 30*, 739–751.
54. Perrin, G. M., & Pierce, I. R. (1959). Psychosomatic aspects of cancer; a review. *Psychosomatic Medicine, 21*, 397–421.

55. Locke, S. E., & Gorman, J. R. (1989). Behavior and immunity. In H. I. Kaplan & B. J. Sadock (Eds.), *Comprehensive textbook of psychiatry*. Williams & Wilkins.
56. Kaplan, H. I., & Sadock, B. J. (1988). *Synopsis of psychiatry* (5th ed., p. 100). Williams & Wilkins.
57. Seligman, M. (1998). *Learned optimism*. Pocket Books.
58. Terman, L., & Oden, M. H. (1947). *The gifted child grows up: Twenty-five years' follow-up of a superior group (genetic studies of genius)*. Standford University Press.
59. Terman, L. M., & Oden, M. H. (1959). *Genetic studies of genius: The gifted group at mid-life; thirty-five years' follow-up of the superior child* (Vol. 5). Stanford University Press.
60. Duckworth, A., Peterson, C., Matthews, M. D., et al. (2007). Grit: Perseverance and passion for long-term goals. *Journal of Personality and Social Psychology, 92*, 1087–1101.
61. Forney, D. S., Wallace-Schutzman, F., & Wiggers, T. T. (1982). Burnout among career development professionals: Preliminary findings and implications. *Personnel and Guidance J, 60*, 435–439.
62. Eldridge, W., Blostein, S., & Richardson, V. (1983). A multidimensional model for assessing factors associated with burnout in human service organizations. *Public Personnel Management, 12*, 315.
63. Gillespie, D. F. (1980). Correlates for active and passive types of burnout. *Journal of Social Service Research, 81*, 1–16.
64. Grimberg, A., DiVall, S. A., Polychronakos, C., et al. (2016). Guidelines for growth hormone and insulin-like growth factor-I treatment in children and adolescents: Growth hormone deficiency, idiopathic short stature, and primary insulin-like growth factor-I deficiency. *Hormone Research in Pædiatrics, 86*(6), 361–397.
65. Antoniazzi, F., Cavarzere, P., & Gaudino, R. (2015). Growth hormone and early treatment. *Minerva Endocrinologica, 40*(2), 129–143.
66. Shochat, T., Haimov, I., & Lavie, P. (1998). Melatonin—The key to the gate of sleep. *Annals of Medicine, 30*, 109–114.
67. Tzischinsky, O., & Lavie, P. (1994). Melatonin possesses a hypnotic effect which is time-dependent. *Sleep, 17*, 638.
68. Roach, G. D., Reid, K. J., Ferguson, S., et al. (2006). The relationship between the rate of melatonin excretion and sleep consolidation for locomotive engineers in natural sleep settings. *Journal of Circadian Rhythms, 18*(4), 8.
69. Hillman, D. R., & Lack, L. C. (2013). Public health implications of sleep loss: The community burden. *Medical Journal of Australia, 199*(S8), S7–S10.
70. Philip, P., Chaufton, C., Orriols, L., et al. (2014). Complaints of poor sleep and risk of traffic accidents: A population-based case-control study. *PLoS ONE, 9*, Article e114102.
71. Czeisler, C. A., Wickwire, E. M., Barger, L. K., et al. (2016). Sleep-deprived motor vehicle operators are unfit to drive: A multidisciplinary expert consensus statement on drowsy driving. *Sleep Health, 2*, 94–99.
72. Gardiner, C., Weakley, J., Burke, L. M., et al. (2025). The effect of alcohol on subsequent sleep in healthy adults: A systematic review and meta-analysis. *Sleep Medicine Reviews, 80*, 1–15.
73. Roehrs, T., & Roth, T. (2001). Sleep, sleepiness, and alcohol use. *Alcohol Research & Health, 25*, 101–109.
74. Ebrahim, I. O., Shapiro, C. M., Williams, A. J., et al. (2013). Alcohol and sleep: effects on normal sleep. *Alcohol, Clinical and Experimental Research, 37*, 539–549.
75. Boyce, R., Glasgow, S. D., Williams, S., et al. (2016). Causal evidence for the role of REM sleep theta rhythm in contextual memory consolidation. *Science, 352*, 812–816.
76. Galbiati, A., Sforza, M., Fasiello, E., et al. (2020). The association between emotional dysregulation and REM sleep features in insomnia disorder. *Brain and Cognition, 146*, Article 105642. https://doi.org/10.1016/j.bandc.2020.105642
77. Oelke, M., De Wachter, S., Drake, M. J., et al. (2017). A practical approach to the management of nocturia. *International Journal of Clinical Practice, 71*, Article e13027.
78. Wahl, S., Engelhardt, M., Schaupp, P., et al. (2019). The inner clock—Blue light sets the human rhythm. *Journal of Biophotonics, 12*, Article e201900102.

79. Bartrop, R. W., Luckhurst, E., Lazarus, L., et al. (1977). Depressed lymphocyte function after bereavement. *Lancet, 1*, 834–836.
80. Irwin, M., Daniels, M., Risch, S., et al. (1988). Plasma cortisol and natural killer cell activity during bereavement. *Biological Psychiatry, 24*, 173–178.
81. Gerra, G., Monti, D., Panerai, A., et al. (2003). Long-term immune-endocrine effects of bereavement: Relationships with anxiety levels and mood. *Psychiatry Research, 121*, 145–158.
82. Buckley, T., Sunari, D., Marshall, A., et al. (2012). Physiological correlates of bereavement and the impact of bereavement interventions. *Dialogues in Clinical Neuroscience, 14*, 129–139.

Part II
Special Resilience-Enhancing Approaches

Chapter 4
Cognitive Behavioral Approach for Managing Stress

4.1 What is Cognitive Behavioral Approach?

Cognitive behavioral approach (CBA) is a type of psychotherapy that aims to modify cognitive distortions by using cognitive and behavioral techniques [1], thereby enhancing resilience.

CBA is a relatively short-term form of psychotherapy that is active and directive, and involves close collaboration between clients and therapists. The two core elements of this approach are the collaborative relationship between clients and therapists and the promotion of self-management [2].

4.2 The Goal of CBA

The primary goal of CBA is to help clients uncover cognitive distortions and ultimately transform maladaptive assumptions. CBA does not aim to cure but to support clients in developing more effective coping strategies for managing stress [2].

4.3 Rationale for the Application of CBA in Coping with Stress

The rationale for applying CBA to cope with stress is as follows:

First, because cognitive patterns shape how stress is experienced, subjective perception has a greater influence on stress severity than the actual events themselves [3]. What is meaningful to one person may hold little significance for another. The impact of a stressful life event depends on the meaning it has for the individual [3, 4].

K. B. Koh, *Body, Mind and Spirituality*, https://doi.org/10.1007/978-3-032-11214-9_4

Second, the cognitive processes that individuals use to cope with stress significantly influence how they experience and interpret stress [5]. In other words, cognitive processes can lead to either effective or ineffective coping, which may ultimately influence health or illnesses.

4.4 Principle of CBA

Clients under stress may have a limited understanding of their problems and may perceive one possible solution. Therefore, clients must first acknowledge their problems and be willing to address them [6]. Problem-solving is viewed as a form of self-control training, where clients first develop general problem-solving skills and then apply them to specific problems [5].

4.4.1 Cognitive Distortions and Maladaptive Assumptions

CBA primarily focuses on identifying and addressing negative cognitive distortions. Cognitive distortions often stem from irrational beliefs (schemas) or maladaptive assumptions (hypotheses). Schemas are often formed in early childhood and may be influenced by factors such as family, religion, society, culture, or the legal system. Addressing underlying schemas or assumptions often leads to more lasting and effective change than focusing solely on surface-level cognitive distortions [2]. Cognitive distortions often emerge when an external event activates a particular schema. For example, a client who responds to criticism from a superior, thinking "I am good for nothing," may hold a maladaptive assumption such as "I must always be perfect to get recognition."

4.4.2 Common Distorted Cognitions

Common distorted cognitions are as follows [2]:

1. All-or-nothing thinking: The tendency to evaluate performance or personal qualities in black-and-white categories.
2. Selective abstraction or attention: Focusing selectively on one or a few pieces of evidence that support their negative ideas, while ignoring all other relevant information.
3. Overgeneralization: Drawing broad conclusions based on a single negative event, assuming it will happen repeatedly.
4. Catastrophizing: Exaggerating potential consequences of difficulties, often leading to constant fear of catastrophic outcomes.

5. Arbitrary inference: Jumping to a negative conclusion without sufficient evidence or facts.
6. Magnification: Magnifying imperfections to the extent that one is likely to think that they are inadequate and inferior to others.
7. "Should" statements: Using rigid rules or expectations that can generate guilt and resentment.
8. Labeling: Personal labeling involves creating a negative identity based on one's errors and imperfections.
9. Emotional reasoning: Believing that one's feelings reflect reality and treating emotions as evidence of how things really are (for example, "I feel inadequate; therefore, I must be a worthless person.").
10. Personalization: taking responsibility for events unrelated to oneself or outside one's control, and interpreting them in a personally meaningful way.

4.4.3 Format of CBA

CBA is a time-limited intervention, typically lasting 15–25 weeks, with sessions held once per week [7].

4.5 The Process of CBA

4.5.1 Cognitive Approach

The cognitive approach includes (1) identifying automatic thoughts and underlying maladaptive assumptions, (2) testing automatic thoughts and maladaptive assumptions, (3) applying cognitive challenges, (4) generating alternatives and reattribution, (5) using self-instruction, and (6) applying new, adaptive assumptions [7].

Identifying Automatic Thoughts and Underlying Maladaptive Assumptions

1. Identifying Automatic Thoughts

For example, after being rejected by a woman, a client may believe that women dislike him.

In such a case, the client may be asked to collect specific data in the form of a diary (self-monitoring), frequency count, or psychological tools such as sentence completion test (SCT) [8] to identify and quantify problematic thoughts.

2. Identifying Maladaptive Assumptions

These assumptions are not conscious thoughts [9]. Examples include "In order to be happy, I must be perfect" or "If anyone doesn't like me, I'm not lovable." Such assumptions often lead to disappointment, failure, and ultimately to depression [7].

3. Self-Monitoring

Self-monitoring strategies are often assigned as homework to help clients identify and assess specific cognitions, particularly in conjunction with hypothesis testing [5]. Clients are taught to monitor their responses to stressors with the aim of identifying patterns in covert and overt events that precede, accompany, and follow stressful experiences. These patterns include cognitive distortions and maladaptive assumptions. Therapists should encourage clients to record their feelings, thoughts, and behaviors before, during, and after stressful events. As clients become familiar with this self-monitoring, therapists assist them in identifying relationships among situational variables, thoughts, and emotional, behavioral, and symptomatic responses [10].

An Example of Self-Monitoring

The severity of emotions is rated from 1 to 100, and the degree of belief in the client's thoughts rated from 1 to 100%.

Date: September 18
Situation (event): Suddenly another car passed by my car on the expressway
Feeling: "This is crazy!" Anger (90)
Thought: "He will someday have a big accident." (90%)
Reaction or Coping: "I will keep distance from other cars." Deep breath
Outcome: Anger (30), initial thought (60%)

Following the coping strategy, the client's anger level decreased from 90 to 30, and the degree of belief in the initial negative thought diminished from 90 to 60%.

Testing Automatic Thoughts and Maladaptive Assumptions

1. Testing Automatic Thoughts

The goal is to help clients reject inaccurate or exaggerated automatic thoughts through careful examination [7]. For example, the therapist might propose the hypothesis, "Your automatic response to any encounter with another person is 'He likes me, he likes me not.'" The collected data will indicate whether the hypothesis should be confirmed, rejected, or modified [5].

2. Testing Maladaptive Assumptions

To test the accuracy of maladaptive assumptions, therapists may ask clients to defend the validity of their assumption. For example, a client may state that he or she should always work up to his or her potential, and a therapist may ask, "Why is that so important to you?" [7]. The client may then adopt and practice specific cognitive and behavioral responses to both anticipated and unexpected stressors [9].

Cognitive Challenges

Many potentially destructive, especially absolutistic cognitions can be logically challenged by providing evidence from the client's own history that contradicts the belief in question. The therapist might offer such a challenge based on his or her knowledge of the client: "You say that you have always been a failure, yet you told me last time that you got promoted.") [5].

Generating Alternatives and Reattributions

1. Generating Alternatives

Once automatic or irrational thoughts have been identified and challenged, the client should generate specific alternative thoughts that are more rational and positive. These alternative thoughts (a more desirable) then replace the original undesirable ones. For example, the idea that "I am a failure at everything that I do" may be replaced with a more balanced thought (a more desirable and less absolute): "Although I did not do well in a certain situation, I have succeeded before and will probably succeed again." [5].

2. Reattributions

Retraining in causal attribution may result in changes in cognitive and behavioral functioning [11, 12]. In general, reattribution focuses on encouraging clients to attribute problematic thoughts or behaviors (e.g., "It's my fault that the team lost") to causes that are personally controllable [5].

Self-Instruction

When cognitions are used to control and direct behavior in an adaptive manner, these cognitions become self-instructions. Thus, the client may overtly or covertly verbalize directions on how to perform the behavior in question [5].

Generalization and Application of New Assumptions

Therapy concludes with the generalization of new underlying assumptions and their application in stressful circumstances [9].

4.5.2 Examples of Interventions [7]

1. Dichotomous thinking: When a client assumes "Everything is either one extreme or another (black or white, good or bad)," the therapist may encourage them to evaluate situations along a continuum.
2. Selective abstraction: When a client assumes "The events that matter are failures," the therapist may use tools such as daily logs (daily records) to help them identify overlooked successes.
3. Overgeneralization: When a client assumes "If it's true in one case, it applies to any case that is even slightly similar," the therapist should expose the faulty logic and help establish criteria for determining degrees of similarity. In cases where the distorted cognition is excessive responsibility, such as "I am responsible for all bad things," the therapist may use reattribution techniques.
4. Catastrophizing: When a client assumes "The worst thing is almost likely to happen to me," the therapist may ask them to calculate the real probabilities and focus on evidence that the worst did not occur.

4.5.3 Techniques for Controlling Thoughts

Several cognitive and behavioral techniques have been designed to control or suppress persistent undesirable thoughts. These techniques do not attempt to challenge or alter the identified thoughts. Such approaches may be useful for obsessive thoughts, which may have already been challenged but still persist. Some techniques for controlling or suppressing thoughts suggested by Shelton and Levy are as follows [13]:

1. Thought stopping: The client is asked to voluntarily produce the unwanted thought, usually aloud, and then the therapist yells, "Stop!," causing the verbalization to cease it immediately. The client is then asked to say "stop" whenever the unwanted thought occurs [14].
2. Changing the environment: The client is asked to leave the room or change activities when the thought occurs.
3. Delaying the thoughts: The client is asked to postpone thinking about the problem for a specified period of time (e.g., delay it for 1.5 h).
4. Implosion (flooding in fantasy) of distressing thoughts: The client is required to repeatedly experience the distressing thought until it no longer triggers emotional arousal. This can be achieved either by repeating the thought aloud or by describing its content. Repetition tends to be more effective for verbal thoughts, while descriptions may be better for recurring visual images.
5. Punishment: The client receives a mild punishment whenever the thoughts occur. As a self-control procedure, the client may slap his or her wrist.
6. Aversive tasks: The client is instructed to perform an aversive task (such as scrubbing the floor) whenever the thought occurs.

7. Redirecting thoughts: The client is asked to redirect the problematic thoughts to a specific time or place (e.g., only allowing the client to worry for 30 min before going to sleep).

4.5.4 Behavioral Approach

Behavioral techniques include scheduling activities, graded task assignments, behavioral rehearsal, self-reliance training, role-playing, diversion, and mastery and pleasure tasks [7].

1. Graded task assignments: To simplify the situation, encourage small accomplishments, and show clients that success is possible, the therapist often breaks the tasks into smaller subtasks.
2. Behavioral rehearsal: Clients imagine and rehearse the specific steps involved in facing and mastering a challenge.
3. Self-reliance training: Clients—especially inpatients—are encouraged to build self-reliance by doing simple tasks such as making their own beds.
4. Role-playing: This is a powerful and useful technique for eliciting automatic thoughts and learning new behaviors.
5. Diversion: It is useful for helping patients cope well during difficult times and includes physical activity, social interaction, work, play, and visual imagery.
6. Mastery and pleasure: Clients are asked to record their daily activities and rate how much mastery and pleasure each activity brings.

Additionally, relaxation methods can also be used to manage anxiety and stress [15].

4.6 Clinical Applications of CBA

CBA has been shown to be effective for individuals with depressive and anxiety disorders [1]. It is also likely to be effective for patients with psychological factors affecting other medical conditions (PFAOMC; previously called psychosomatic disorders) [10, 16].

4.7 Summary

1. Cognitive behavioral approach (CBA) is a type of psychotherapy that aims to modify cognitive distortions through cognitive and behavioral techniques, thereby enhancing resilience.
2. This approach does not aim to cure but to help clients develop more effective coping strategies to deal with stress.

3. The cognitive components include identifying automatic thoughts and underlying maladaptive assumptions, testing automatic thoughts and maladaptive assumptions, cognitive challenges, generating alternatives and reattributions, using self-instruction, and applying new assumptions.
4. Behavioral techniques include scheduling activities, tracking mastery and pleasure, graded task assignments, behavioral rehearsal, self-reliance training, role-playing, and diversion techniques.

References

1. Beck, A. T., & Rush, A. J. (1989). Cognitive therapy. In H. I. Kaplan & B. J. Sadock (Eds.), *Comprehensive textbook of psychiatry* (pp. 1541–1550). Williams & Wilkins.
2. Freeman, A. (1987). Cognitive therapy: An overview. In A. Freeman & V. Greenwood (Eds.), *Cognitive therapy* (pp. 19–35). Human Science Press.
3. Reiser, M. F. (1984). *Mind, brain, body: Toward a convergence of psychoanalysis and neurobiology*. Basic Books, Inc. (pp.164–85).
4. Koh, K. B. (1992). Coping with job stress. *New Med J, 35*, 11–21.
5. Cotton, D. H. G. (1990). *Stress management: An integrated approach to therapy* (pp. 189–213). Brunner.
6. D'Zurilla, T. J., & Goldfried, M. R. (1971). Problem solving and behavior modification. *Journal of Abnormal Psychology, 78*, 107–126.
7. Kaplan, H. I., & Sadock, B. J. (2003). *Synopsis of psychiatry: Behavioral sciences and clinical psychiatry* (pp. 956–960). Lippincott Williams & Wilkins.
8. Koh, K. B. (2011). *Stress and psychosomatic medicine* (2nd ed., pp. 331–340). Ilchokak.
9. Rush, A. J. (1984). Cognitive therapy. In T. B. Karasu (Ed.), *The Psychiatric therapies* (pp. 397–414). American Psychiatric Association.
10. Holroyd, K. A., Appel, M. A., & Andrasik, F. (1983). A cognitive-behavioral approach to psychophysiological disorders. In D. Meichenbaum & M. E. Jaremko (Eds.), *Stress reduction and prevention* (pp. 219–259). Plenum Press.
11. Forsterling, F. (1980). Attributional aspects of cognitive behavior modification: A theoretical approach and suggestions for technique. *Cognitive Therapy and Research, 4*, 27–37.
12. Forsterling, F. (1986). Attributional conceptions in clinical psychology. *American Psychologist, 41*, 275–285.
13. Shelton, J. L., & Levy, R. L. (1981). *Behavioral assignments and treatment compliance*. Research Press.
14. Stern, R. S. (1970). Treatment of a case of obsessional neurosis using thought-stopping technique. *The British Journal of Psychiatry, 117*, 441–442.
15. Goldberg. R. J. (1987). Anxiety in the medically ill. In A. Stoudemire & B. S, Fogel (Eds.), *Principles of medical psychiatry*. Grune & Stratton Inc.
16. Koh, K. B. (1988). Stress perception of patients with psychosomatic disorders. *J Korean Neuropsychiatric Assoc, 27*, 514–523.

Chapter 5
Cognitive Behavioral Approach for Type A Behavior

5.1 Rationale for Cognitive Behavioral Therapy of Type A Behavior

Type A behavior is not only an independent risk factor for coronary heart disease (CHD) [1], but it has also been shown to improve through psychological interventions [2]. The recurrence rate of myocardial infarction has been reduced following the modification of type A behavior [3].

The mechanism of cognitive behavioral therapy for type A behavior involves reducing sympathetic nervous system (SNS) arousal through cognitive and relaxation techniques [4].

5.2 Cognitive Distortions in Type A Behavior

Cognitive distortions commonly observed in individuals with type A behavior include all-or-nothing thinking, selective attention, personalization, and attribution of causality [5].

Type A individuals often express concern that if they say "no" to an opportunity, despite already having too many commitments, they may never get another chance [6].

They also tend to suppress all stimuli unrelated to the task at hand, making them unaware of early symptoms and signs of CHD [7].

Personalization refers to a tendency to exaggerate a sense of self-importance, beyond normal egocentricity [5].

Attributions of causality refer to beliefs about why things happen [8]. For example, type A individuals often attribute success to effort and, when they fail, blame it on not trying hard enough [9].

K. B. Koh, *Body, Mind and Spirituality*, https://doi.org/10.1007/978-3-032-11214-9_5

5.3 Cognitive Behavioral Therapy for Features of Type A Behavior

5.3.1 *Time Urgency*

Interventions for the self-defeating time urgency typical of type A individuals include:

1. Encouraging clients to prioritize daily activities and find a balance between work and relaxation, productivity and play [1].
2. Teaching effective coping methods for job stress, such as relaxation techniques [10].
3. Helping clients shift their attitudes when facing uncontrollable situations. For example, being stuck in traffic may cause less stress if one can reframe it as a normal, uncontrollable event [5].

5.3.2 *Perfectionism*

Due to all-or-nothing thinking, type A individuals often equate mistakes or imperfections with total failure [6]. Interventions for perfectionism include [5]:

1. Helping clients shift their goal from achieving perfection to accepting imperfection.
2. Questioning clients about perfectionistic rituals and their consequences to facilitate attitude change.
3. Encouraging clients to experiment with new behaviors, starting with small, manageable tasks.

5.3.3 *Achievement Striving*

Selective attention enhances achievement striving by suppressing awareness of personal limitations. Interventions aim to help clients recognize information they tend to ignore (i.e., denial). For example, therapists may present the positive and negative consequences of type A behavior [6].

5.3.4 *Excessive Work Involvement*

Type A individuals often attribute outcomes to factors within their control. Interventions should help them distinguish between what can and cannot be controlled, attributing some outcomes to external factors. In cases where job demands are overwhelming, exploring alternative employment options may be necessary [5].

5.3.5 *Low Self-Esteem*

For many type A individuals, self-worth is tied to achievement [5]. This belief means that their self-esteem fluctuates based on accomplishments and external approval [6].

Therapeutic approaches [5] include:

1. Questioning why rejection or criticism feels so threatening.
2. Realistically assessing the consequences of such events.
3. Broadening the sources of self-esteem to include relationships and an unconditional sense of self-worth, aiming to foster a more balanced and stable sense of adequacy.

5.3.6 *Hostility*

In many studies [11–13], hostility and anger were found to play an important role in type A behavior.

Type A individuals often externalize problems and believe others should change [14].

Cognitive behavioral interventions for hostility include:

1. Helping clients find a middle ground between aggression and passivity by discussing assertiveness principles [15].
2. Helping clients identify thoughts that arise during emotional arousal [5].
3. Encouraging clients to challenge irrational thoughts while using relaxation techniques [16].
4. Helping clients address maladaptive assumptions. For example, replacing the belief "others should do things my way" with a more functional alternative such as "everyone has their own way."

It is also helpful to question the expectation that others must change [5].

5.3.7 *Depression*

Many type A individuals believe they must work for their worth. When illness or exhaustion hinders accomplishment, depression may result. Therapy helps clients explore these underlying beliefs and reframe them within the context of their current needs and circumstances. Ultimately, clients are guided to transition from a competitive model of self-worth to a more cooperative one [5].

Case

A 32-year-old male patient visited the department of neurology as an outpatient with symptoms of pressing and paralyzing sensations in the left side of the head. Laboratory findings revealed no abnormalities. A neurological examination and a brain CT did not show abnormalities either. Psychotropics such as amitriptyline, alprazolam, and propranolol were prescribed by the neurologist for nearly 1 year, but no significant improvement was noted. He was therefore referred to the department of psychiatry.

The patient had been working on a joint project with a university professor for 1 year, but the professor gave up midway. At that time, his superior demanded him to complete the unresolved project quickly. He struggled to complete the project and eventually failed. After that, he started to experience intolerable headaches.

During the first interview, the patient was somewhat talkative, anxious, and very tense, complaining of a pressing sensation in the left side of his head. He also showed suppressed anger and hostility toward his superior. His somatic symptoms such as the paralyzing sensation in the left side of his head and the headache were aggravated by stressors at work.

A combined diagnosis of migraine and tension headache was made. The main stressors exacerbating his somatic symptoms were found to be associated with his work overload and his relationship with his superior. In a series of interviews, his cognitive distortions in relation to these stressors were observed repetitively.

His depressive mood and headache became more severe after he was blamed for his poor job performance and his demand for going abroad was rejected. In a self-assessment statement, he described, "I was severely scolded for having ordered another staff to do my job. I felt very bad when the superior shouted at me over trivial things. At that time, I got a severe headache and felt like a fool when I didn't say anything while being scolded. I wondered if the superior looked down on me or if I was incompetent." He said, "to other staff, he would not do the same. In spite of my effort, he doesn't seem to trust me at all." As mentioned above, the patient tended to show cognitive distortions such as magnification and selective abstraction. In addition, he showed arbitrary inference, saying "I don't have any prospects in the future at all."

In the relationship with his subordinates, he also showed such cognitive distortions. He was very angry when a subordinate was absent from work without asking for a leave. At that time, he experienced a pressing and stiffening sensation of the head, thought that he was really incompetent, and wondered if he was looked down on. In addition, he showed mislabeling ("I am stupid") and 'should' statements ("My subordinates should always wait for me; I should command them as their head.").

Maladaptive assumptions seen in this patient were personal ("I must be perfect to be successful and happy") and related to his family and work ("I [or subordinates] should be obedient to seniors [or superiors]."). His statements showed no midway between 100% right and 100% wrong. The therapist tried to make him perceive different degrees of severity in these thoughts as well as in his mood and his headache, by using self-assessment techniques.

As an example, the patient got promoted to section head through fierce competition. The therapist thus pointed out to the patient that this event did not prove his dichotomous thinking, such as "my superior does not trust me at all," but posed a direct challenge to his cognitive distortions. He was also recommended to practice self-assertion when being treated unfairly by his superior.

The patient thought that his superior did not trust him at all when he was scolded, but the next day the superior felt sorry for his behavior and the patient realized that the superior did not always hate him. During the therapeutic sessions, he was allowed to self-assert and to find alternatives for coping with stress. For example, he was recommended to do pleasurable activities outside of work. He thus started to play tennis after work and to learn how to swim. On weekends, he went hiking or bowling with his wife.

Thereafter, even though the patient still complained of his dissatisfaction toward his superior, the frequency of his thoughts of always being scolded and unfairly treated was markedly reduced. Even when he talked about the superior, he was no longer serious or depressed and the severity and frequency of his headache was also diminished. In addition, he showed significant changes in his behavior; he went to his superior and complained to him about his transfer to another section.

The following are extracts from the patient's self-assessments during the therapeutic sessions.

*The severity of emotions and symptoms is rated from 1 to 100, and the degree of belief in the patient's thoughts rated from 1 to 100%.

Date: August 28
Situation (event): My request for going abroad was rejected by the director.
Feeling: Depressed (50), pressing sensation of the head and headache (70)
Thought: I probably made a bad impression on the superior (80%)
Reaction or Coping: Busy schedule along with the company's education program, so gave up going abroad and decided to focus on the education program.
Outcome: Depressed (30), pressing sensation of the head and headache (30), initial thought (40%)

Date: September 7
Situation (event): My subordinates were supposed to play tennis with me but left before I got there.
Feeling: A feeling of betrayal (70)
Thought: They seem to ignore me (70%), I am personally inadequate (60%).
Reaction or Coping: Am I reacting too sensitively? I can play tennis with others instead
Outcome: A sense of betrayal (40), initial thought (50%)

Date: September 17
Situation (event): One of my subordinates was absent from work without notice.

Feeling: Angry (70 ~ 80), pressing and stiff sensation of the head (70 ~ 80)
Thought: Am I incompetent? (70%).
Reaction or Coping: I won't forgive him if he behaves like this one more time. I will ask him to submit a reason for his absence.
Outcome: Angry (30), pressing and stiff sensation of the head (50), initial thought (30%)

In this case, it took a long time for such a therapy to have an effect on the patient's headache symptoms, because long-term assessments were needed to understand his problems objectively. Moreover, it was not easy to alter the patient's coping methods, because of his rigid and inflexible personality along with various interpersonal conflicts.

5.4 Summary

1. Common cognitive distortions in type A behavior include all-or-nothing thinking, selective attention, personalization, and attribution of causality.
2. Cognitive behavioral therapy can be applied to address key features of the type A behavior, such as time urgency, perfectionism, achievement striving, excessive work involvement, low self-esteem, hostility, and depression.
3. Individualized intervention is essential, as the predominant features of type A behavior vary from person to person.

References

1. Haynes, S. G., & Matthews, K. A. (1988). The association of Type A behavior with cardiovascular disease: update and critical review. In B. K. Houston & C. R. Snyder (Eds.), *Type A behavior pattern research, theory and intervention.* Wiley.
2. Bennett, P., & Carroll, D. (1990). Stress management approaches to the prevention of heart disease. *British Journal of Clinical Psychology, 29*, 1–12.
3. Friedman, M., Thorensen, C. E., Gill, J. J., et al. (1986). Alteration of type A behavior and its effect on cardiac recurrences in postmyocardial infarction patients: Summary of the recurrent coronary prevention project. *American Heart Journal, 112*, 653–665.
4. Suinn, R. M., & Bloom, L. J. (1978). Anxiety management training for pattern A behavior. *Journal of Behavioral Medicine, 1*, 25–35.
5. Kinchla, J. (1987). Cognitive approaches to management of the type A behavior pattern. In A. Freeman & V. Greenwood (Eds.), *Cognitive therapy: Application in psychiatric and medical settings* (pp. 162–182). Human Sciences Press.
6. Price, V. A. (1982). *Type A behavior pattern.* Academic Press.
7. Matthews, K. A., & Brunson, B. I. (1979). Allocation of attention and the type A coronary-prone behavior pattern. *J Per Soc Psychol, 37*, 2081–2090.
8. Kelley, H. H. (1967). Attribution theory in social psychology. In D. Levine (Ed.), *Nebraska symposium on motivation* (pp. 192–238). University of Nebraska Press.

9. Margolis, L. H., McLeroy, K. R., Runyan, C. W., et al. (1983). Type A behavior: An ecological approach. *J Beh Med, 6*, 245–258.
10. Burman, M. A., Pennebaker, J. W., & Glass, D. C. (1975). Time consciousness, achievement striving and the type A coronary prone behavior pattern. *Journal of Abnormal Psychology, 84*, 76–79.
11. Chesney, M. A., Hecker, M. A., & Black, G. W. (1988). Coronary-prone behavior in the WCGS: A new methodology. In B. K. Houston & C. R. Snyder (Eds.), *Type A behavior pattern: Research, theory and intervention.* Wiley.
12. Matthews, K. A., Glass, D. C., Rosenman, R. H., et al. (1977). Competitive drive, pattern A, and coronary heart disease: A further analysis of some data from the western collaborative group study. *Journal of Chronic Diseases, 30*, 489–498.
13. Dembroski, T. M., & Costa, P. T. (1988). Assessment of coronary prone behavior: A current overview. *Annals of Behavioral Medicine, 10*, 60–70.
14. Powell, L. (1983). Workshop on the type A behavior pattern. Presented at society for behavioral medicine convention.
15. Kiester, E. (1984). The use of anger. *Psychology Today, 18*, 26.
16. Ellis, R. A., & Harper, R. A. (1975). New guide to rational living. Wilshire Book Co.

Chapter 6
The Role of Religion and Spirituality in Body and Mind

6.1 What is Religion and Spirituality?

Religion can be described as a set of beliefs about the transcendent shared by a community [1, 2]. Spirituality can be characterized as an individual's relationship with and experience of the transcendent [1].

6.2 Spirituality as Coping with Stress

Religious cognition and behavior can help effectively deal with stressful events and conditions [3]. Spirituality plays a buffering role in the face of negative life events [4–8]. In addition, spirituality can be positively viewed as enhancing one's hope and confidence [5, 9].

6.3 Effects of Religious Coping

6.3.1 Self-Esteem or Personal Efficacy

In previous research, religious involvement (e.g., religious attendance and private piety) was positively associated with self-esteem and personal efficacy [10, 11].

K. B. Koh, *Body, Mind and Spirituality*, https://doi.org/10.1007/978-3-032-11214-9_6

6.3.2 Physical and Mental Health

Religious cognitions and behaviors such as prayer, meditation, and other devotional pursuits are likely to help effectively deal with serious health problems and bereavement [3, 12, 13]. People who profess stronger spiritual beliefs seem to resolve their grief more rapidly and completely after the death of a close person than those with no spiritual beliefs [14]. In addition, religion/spirituality is associated with reduced depression and anxiety and increased longevity [15–17].

6.3.3 Feelings of Control and Confidence

Some coping styles such as collaboration with a divine other can enhance feelings of control and confidence in the ability to manage difficult and stressful situations and produce desirable health outcomes [7, 18].

6.3.4 Adjustment of Self-Concept

Religion can help individuals adjust their self-concept so that physical problems are less threatening to their personal identity [12].

6.3.5 Reassessment of the Meaning of Stressful Conditions

Religious cognitions and behaviors such as prayers and scripture readings may change primary appraisals (i.e., evaluating whether a stressor is threatening or not, followed by anxiety), leading to reassessing the meaning of stressful conditions as opportunities for spiritual growth or learning, or as part of a broader divine plan rather than as a challenge to personal identity [19].

However, religious coping styles such as passively leaving responsibility for resolving crises entirely up to divine intervention are likely to yield poor health [3].

Case

This is the author's personal experience while struggling with prostate cancer.

I had benign prostate hypertrophy (BPH) for more than 20 years and had taken medications such as Harnal (tamsulosin hydrochloride). First, the level of prostate-specific antigen (PSA) notably increased from 3.9 ng/ml to 4.6 ng/ml, then six months later to 6.2 ng/ml. Consequently, Magnetic Resonance Imaging (MRI) was done, showing findings suggestive of cancer, and a tissue biopsy was performed, which revealed prostate cancer with a high level of malignancy (Gleason level 4 or 5).

Therefore, I had to undergo a Positron Emission Tomography (PET) scan to check if the cancer spread to bones or not. I felt very anxious the day before the scan was performed. Then, I prayed, "God, please give me a courageous mind to accept whatever the results of the scan are."

After this prayer, I could get my mind back on the track. I stayed calm during the PET scan. Fortunately, the results did not reveal bone metastases. I then received anti-testosterone hormone therapy after prostate cancer was confirmed. Thereafter, the PSA levels markedly decreased. However, I often experienced urgency and middle insomnia (frequent awakening).

During this difficult period, I often had to practice as an actor in an upcoming musical. I was happy to have finished the musical five times for four days without giving up. I really enjoyed the musical performances. Prior to admission, two ministers of my church prayed and promised that they would pray for me daily.

On the upper part of the entrance to the operating room and on the ceiling of the room, some brief Bible verse was noticed: "Do not fear, for I am with you" (Isaiah 41:10).

Finally, with a calm mind I successfully underwent an operation for the cancer.

After the operation, I had terrible experiences of being in low spirits because of poor appetite and urinary incontinence. In particular, my poor appetite made me feel pessimistic. I wondered what living like this meant. Thereafter, I felt grateful for eating well. Fortunately, I have made a nearly complete recovery from this suffering.

6.4 Religious Involvement and Mental and Physical Well-Being

6.4.1 Emotions and Physiological Responses

Religious involvement may lead to positive emotions such as forgiveness [20], contentment, and love, as well as negative emotions such as guilt andfear. These emotions may affect physiological functions through psychoneuro immunological or neuroendocrine pathways, leading to alterations in health status [15].

6.4.2 Regulation of Health-Related Behaviors

Religious involvement, especially participation in religious communities, may promote mental and physical well-being by regulating health-related behaviors in ways that decrease the risk of diseases. This includes 1) discouraging behaviors that increase the risk of health problems, and 2) encouraging positive and low-stress lifestyle choices. Actually, religious involvement is inversely associated with alcohol, tobacco, and substance use and abuse [21, 22].

6.4.3 *Religious Involvement and Self-Perception*

Religious involvement may promote better health by enhancing feelings of self-esteem or a sense of intrinsic moral self-worth, feelings of efficacy, or the perception that one can control one's personal affairs; promoting constructive coping responses; and enhancing social support [15].

How might religious involvement enhance the important dimensions of self-perception? Through devotional activities (e.g., prayer and scriptural studies), individuals may construct personal relationships with a divine other [23, 24]. Individuals may gain a sense of self-worth and control by developing a close personal relationship with a potent divine other who unconditionally loves and cares for each person and engages interactively in a quest for solace and guidance. They may also enjoy a sense of vicarious control over their affairs through their alliance with an omniscient and omnipotent deity (e.g., with God, all things are possible) [25].

6.5 Spirituality and Social Support

Spirituality (e.g., sharing religious thoughts and insights and praying for others) [26, 27] is a source of social support [28]. Shared values within religious communities may provide a set of shared meanings concerning human suffering, adjustment, and support [27, 29].

6.6 Role of Religion and Spirituality in Depression of the Medically Ill

Religious beliefs and behaviors help manage emotional distress [30–33]. Religious involvement helps older people with chronic medical problems cope better with these conditions and may protect them from depression [34]. Depressed older inpatients with heart failure or chronic pulmonary disease who have a strong personal religious commitment and intrinsic motivation are likely to remit more quickly from depression after hospital discharge [35].

Religion may give patients a sense of purpose and meaning in life despite health problems [36], provide hope and optimism about the future [37], and increase their sense of control (through prayer) [38]. In addition, religion may enhance social support outside their immediate family. These effects enable older patients to cope better with their illnesses [39].

In particular, among outpatients with heart failure, greater spiritual well-being, particularly meaning/peace, was strongly associated with lower levels of depression. This result suggests that the enhancement of patients' sense of spiritual well-being might reduce or prevent depression, and thus improve their quality of life [40].

However, religion may increase guilt and neurosis [41] when it often stigmatizes depression, or subtle messages may be promoted by religious groups that depression is due to a lack of faith [35].

Depressed patients who are not religious may be at greater risk for persistent depression. Nonetheless, encouraging such patients to become more religiously involved is inappropriate because no research shows positive findings such as mental health benefits in those becoming religious for mental health reasons alone [35].

However, whether religiously inclined or not, clinicians need to view a religious community as a potential source of support and healing, especially for severely ill patients who have few other options [35].

6.7 Practical Application of Spirituality in Terminally Ill Patients

Addressing spiritual needs of the dying is generally neglected in palliative care practice [42]. However, individuals may have greater spiritual needs during terminal illness. Therefore, addressing the spiritual needs of these patients may help enhance their recovery from illnesses [16].

Generally, religion or spirituality plays a positive role in patients coping with illnesses such as cancer [43–45]. Life-threatening illnesses such as cancer can be stimuli for the expansion of one's previous concepts of self-boundaries, leading to changes in personallife purpose and meaning. Therefore, the diagnosis of a terminal illness may be regarded as either a crisis or an opportunity for growth and meaning, as one learns to cope with it [37].

In one study, the degree of meaning/peace was negatively associated with the levels of depression in terminal patients with cancer [43]. In contrast, depression and hopelessness were associated with poorer survival in cancer patients [46]. Therefore, addressing depression, hopelessness, and loss of meaning in the treatment of terminally ill patients is important [47].

6.8 Assessment of Spiritual Beliefs

An assessment of spiritual beliefs can be performed using questions regarding faith, importance, community, and how to address "The FICA spiritual history" [48].

6.8.1 Faith

Do you have a religious faith? Do you consider yourself spiritual?

6.8.2 *Importance*

How important are your religious beliefs and spirituality and how might they influence decisions related to your health?

6.8.3 *Community*

Are you part of a religious, spiritual, or other community (e.g., a member of a church)? If so, how does this community support you?

6.8.4 *How to Address*

How might I address your spiritual needs?

6.8.5 *Other Questions*

The following questions can also help physicians recognize the spiritual needs of patients: "What meaning does this illness have for you?" "What helps you overcome tough times?" "To whom do you turn when you need support?" "What are your hopes, expectations, and fears regarding the future?" [49, 50].

For terminally ill patients, spiritual history is regarded as a crucial component of palliative medicine [51–53]. This spiritual assessment can help clinicians learn how religion affects patients' abilities to cope with illnesses, social support, and medical decisions [54]

6.9 Care of the Terminally Ill

A combination of science and art, such as medicine and psychiatry, is essential for the care of terminally ill patients. The art often depends on the caregiver's personality, the past history of the patient and family, and their psychosocial values and issues [55].

Psychiatric consultations can be beneficial in the care of patients with terminal cancer and their families because conflicts may arise regardingcare decisions [56]. Such consultants should address a variety of issues in the care of patients: the patient's and family's understanding of terminal illness, cultural or religious mindset, family functioning (cohesion), family resources (e.g., social support, physical and psychological stamina, and financial support), and the family's open communication [56].

Treatment for the terminally ill is aimed at providing maximal comfort during their remaining lifespan.

Therapists need to make patients and family members aware that the person who is dying has not changed; only their life expectancy has changed and their emotional needs may intensify [56].

6.10 Principles of Interventions for Spiritual Suffering at the End of Life

Support from those close to the patients and religion may play a crucial role in their coping with the process of dying during the terminal stage [57]. Psychotherapeutic interventions for the spiritual suffering of patients with terminal illnesses aim to improve spiritual well-being and a sense of meaning while diminishing hopelessness, demoralization, and distress during end-of-life care [58].

Individual and group psychotherapies are used as interventions for patients with cancer. However, group psychotherapy may be more effective thanindividual psychotherapy for these patients [58]. This is because, unlike individual psychotherapy, group psychotherapy will help patients cope better with their conditions by providing opportunities to share their personal experiences together and support them.

A step-by-step therapeutic approach to spiritual suffering is as follows [47]:

1. Controlling physical symptoms
2. Providing a supportive presence
3. Encouraging life review to assist in recognizing the purpose, value, and meaning of life
4. Exploring guilt, forgiveness, and reconciliation
5. Facilitating religious expressions
6. Reframing goals
7. Encouraging meditation
8. Focusing on healing (reduction of distress) rather than cure (removal of causes).

This kind of psychotherapy utilizes the concept of self-transcendence (i.e., expansion of personal boundaries) and meaning, as developed by Victor Frankl [59–62]. Self-transcendence is an aspect of logotherapy that enables one to have a sense of meaning and purpose in life [37]. The word "logo" is derived from the Greek "logos," which indicates "meaning."

In particular, spiritual care from the medical system helps patients transition to hospice care and improves their well-being near death. Furthermore, spiritual support may reduce the risk of aggressive interventions (sometimes unproven) at the end of life [63].

Promoting religion to deal with spiritual concerns or end-of-life suffering is not recommended for all patients. However, interventions based on the "meaning" component of spirituality are likely to be more universally applicable to patients and accepted by health care providers as well as patients [37].

Clinicians can play a crucial role in spiritual assessments and making pastoral care referrals. The need for education of physicians on spiritual care and the importance of integrating pastoral care into multidisciplinary medical teams will be more emphasized in the future [63].

The patient's own minister can help the patient and family reduce their distress by softening the dying process [64].

6.11 Meaning-Centered Psychotherapy for Advanced Cancer Patients [37]

Meaning-centered group psychotherapy for patients with advanced cancer uses Frankl's concept of logotherapy (meaning and spirituality). The premise of logotherapy is that failure to find meaning in life results in psychological distress.

This therapy is designed to help patients with advanced cancer sustain or enhance their sense of meaning, peace, and purpose in their lives. Individual logotherapy for patients with terminal illnesses needs six 45-min sessions over a 2-week period. The session themes include: for example, (1) cancer and meaning; (2) meaning of life; (3) life projects; (4) limitations and finiteness of life; (5) responsibility and deeds; (6) experience, nature, art, humor; and (7) hopes for the future.

A logotherapist helps patients discover who they are, how they wish to interpret their present situation, and what they want to become.

Importance is placed on an individual's acceptance of the freedom to change their attitude toward the difficulties experienced, develop a new perspective on their identity, and reinterpret the significance of their life's contributions positively.

The steps undertaken include: (1) eliciting sources (e.g., activities and relationships) that provide meaning in each patient's life; (2) focusing on the impact of illness; (3) dealing with the fear of dying using the technique of dereflection (i.e., directing a person's attention away from their problem and toward something important to the person); and (4) enhancing a sense of closure with significant others in life as death approaches.

Meaning-centered psychotherapy can change a man with old views to one with new views or perspectives on their life.

6.12 Serenity Prayer

The "Serenity Prayer" by Reinhold Niebuhr may help us cope with difficult situations and serious health problems.

"God, grant me the serenity to accept the things I cannot change,
the courage to change the things I can,
and the wisdom to know the difference."

The serenity prayer helps us acknowledge that some things in life are beyond our control. When we recognize that something is beyond our control, we are free to stop trying to change it. Fighting futile battles is exhausting and stressful. This encourages constructive action to direct our lives in positive ways with courage (the help of God), even though it is not easy to change something in our lives.

As a result, knowing the difference between the two is important to avoid spending our energy on things that we cannot change. Whenever we face difficult things in life, it is important to reflect on what we need to accept—things that we cannot change in contrast to things that can be changed, even though they require courage [65].

6.13 Summary

1. Religious cognitions and behaviors effectively deal with stressful events.
2. Religious involvement may promote better health by enhancing feelings of self-esteem, efficacy, or perception of control; promoting constructive coping; and enhancing social support.
3. Participation in religious communities may promote mental and physical well-being by regulating health-related behaviors.
4. Spirituality such as praying for others is a source of social support.
5. Religion/spirituality is associated with reduced depression and anxiety, and increased longevity.
6. Religion/spirituality may give depressed patients with physical diseases a sense of purpose and meaning in life despite their health problems.
7. Meaning-centered group psychotherapy may help patients with advanced cancer search for meaning and purpose and enhance a sense of peace in their lives
8. Clinicians can play a crucial role in spiritual assessment and making pastoral care referrals.

References

1. Sulmasy, D. P. (2007). *The Rebirth of the clinic: An introduction to spirituality in health care.* Georgetown University Press.

2. Koenig, H. G. (2008). *Medicine, religion, and health: Where science and spirituality meet.* Templeton Foundation Press.
3. Pargament, K. I. (1997). *The psychology of religion and coping.* Guilford.
4. Crawford, M., Handal, P., & Weiner, R. (1989). The relationship between religion and mental health/distress. *Review of Religious Research, 31*, 16–22.
5. Ellison, C. (1991). Religious involvement and subjective well-being. *Journal of Health and Social Behavior, 32*, 80–99.
6. Hathaway, W., & Pargament, K. (1990). Intrinsic religiousness, religious coping, and psychosocial competence: A covariance structural anaylsis. *Journal of Scientific Study of Religion, 29*, 423–441.
7. Pargament, K., Kennell, J., Hathaway, W., et al. (1988). Religion and the problem-solving process: Three styles of coping. *Journal of Scientific Study of Religion, 27*, 90–104.
8. Ross, C. (1990). Religion and psychological distress. *Journal of Scientific Study of Religion, 29*, 235–245.
9. Maton, R. (1987). Spiritual discernment in psychiatric patients. *Journal of Religion and Health, 26*, 125–130.
10. Bergin, A. E. (1983). Religiosity and mental health: A critical reevaluation and meta-analysis. *Professional Psychology: Research and Practice., 14*, 170–184.
11. Gartner, J. D., Larson, D. B., & Allen, G. D. (1991). Religious commitment and mental health: A review of the empirical literature. *Journal of Psychology and Theology, 19*, 6–25.
12. Idler, E. L. (1995). Religion, health, and non-physical senses of self. *Social Forces, 74*, 683–704.
13. Mattlin, J. A., Wethington, E., & Kessler, R. C. (1990). Situational determinants of coping and coping effectiveness. *Journal of Health and Social Behavior, 31*, 103–122.
14. Walsh, K., King, M., Jones, L., et al. (2002). Spiritual beliefs may affect outcome of bereavement: Prospective study. *BMJ, 324*, 1551–1556.
15. Ellison, C. G., & Levin, J. S. (1998). The religion-health connection: Evidence, theory, and future directions. *Health Education & Behavior, 25*, 700–720.
16. Mueller, P. S., Plevak, D. J., & Rummans, T. A. (2001). Religious involvement, spirituality, and medicine: Implications for clinical practice. *Mayo Clinic Proceedings, 76*, 1225–1235.
17. Matthews, D. A., McCullough, M. E., Larson, D. B., et al. (1998). Religious commitment and health status: A review of the research and implications for family medicine. *Archives of Family Medicine, 7*, 118–124.
18. Pargament, K., Ensing, D. S., & Falgout, K. et al. (1990). God help me: (1) religious coping efforts as predictors of the outcomes to significant negative life events. *American Journal of Community* Psychology, *18*, 793–824.
19. Foley, D. P. (1988). Eleven interpretations of personal suffering. *J Religion Health, 27*, 321–328.
20. Kaplan, B. H., Monroe-Blum, H., & Blazer, D. G. (1994). Religion, health, and forgiveness: Traditions and challenges. In J. S. Levin (Ed.), *Religion in aging and health: Theoretical foundations and methodological frontiers* (pp. 52–77). Sage.
21. Cochran, J. K., Beeghley, L., & Bock, E. W. (1988). Religiosity and alcohol behavior: An exploration of reference group theory. *Sociological Forum, 3*, 256–276.
22. Koenig, H. G., George, L. K., Meador, K. G., et al. (1994). Religious practices and alcoholism in a Sothern adult population. *Hospital & Community Psychiatry, 45*, 225–231.
23. Pollner, M. (1989). Divine relations, social relations, and well-being. *Journal of Health and Social Behavior, 30*, 92–104.
24. Ellison, C. G. (1994). Religion, the life stress paradigm, and the study of depression. In J. S. Levin (Ed.), *Religion in aging and health: Theoretical foundations and methodological frontiers* (pp. 78–121). Sage.
25. Poloma, M. M., & Gallup, G. (1991). *Varieties of prayer: A survey report.* Trinity Press International.
26. Taylor, R. J., & Chatters, L. M. (1988). Church members as a source of informal social support. *Review of Religious Research, 30*, 193–202.
27. Maton, K. I. (1989). Community settings as buffers of life stress? Highly supportive churches, mutual help groups, and senior centers. *American Journal of Commun Psychology, 17*, 203–232.

28. Sullivan, W. P. (1993). It helps me to be a whole person: The role of spirituality among the mentally challenged. *Psychosocial Rehabilitation Journal, 16*, 125–134.
29. Grasmik, H. G., Bursik, R. J., & Cochran, J. K. (1991). Render unto Caesar what is Caesar's: Religiosity and taxpayers' inclinations to cheat. *The Sociological Quarterly, 32*, 251–266.
30. Koenig, H. G., Smiley, M., & Gonzales, J. P. (1988). *Religion, health and aging: A review and theoretical integration* (pp. 13–21). Greenwood Press.
31. Swanson, W. C., & Harter, C. L. (1971). How do elderly blacks cope in New Orleans? *International Journal of Aging and Human Development, 2*, 210–216.
32. Rosen, C. C. (1982). Ethnic differences among impoverished rural elderly in use of religion as a coping mechanism. *Journal of Rural Community Psychology, 3*, 27–34.
33. Conway, K. (1985-1986). Coping with the stress of medical problems among black and white elderly. *International Journal of Aging and Human Development, 21*, 39–48.
34. Sansone, R. A., Khatain, K., & Rodenhauser, P. (1990). The role of religion in psychiatric education: A national survey. *Academic Psychiatry, 14*, 34–38.
35. Koenig, H. G. (2007). Religion and remission of depression in medical inpatients with heart failure/pulmonary disease. *The Journal of Nervous and Mental Disease, 195*, 389–395.
36. George, L. K., Larson, D. B., Koenig, H. G., et al. (2000). Spirituality and health: What we know, what we need to know. *Journal of Social and Clinical Psychology, 19*, 102–116.
37. Breitbart, W. (2002). Spirituality and meaning in supportive care: Spirituality and meaning-centered group psychotherapy interventions in advanced cancer. *Supportive Care in Cancer, 10*, 272–280.
38. Koenig, H. G. (2005). *Faith and mental health*. Templeton Foundation Press.
39. Koenig, H. G. (1998). Religious beliefs and practices of hospitalized medically ill older adults. *International Journal of Geriatric Psychiatry, 13*, 213–224.
40. Bekelman, D. B., et al. (2007). Spiritual well-being and depression in patients with heart failure. *Journal of General Internal Medicine, 22*, 470–477.
41. Freud, S. (1962). Future of an illusion (1927). In J. Stachey (Ed.), *Standard edition of the complete psychological works of Sigmund Freud* (p. 43). Hogarth Press.
42. Kearney, M., & Mount, B. (2000). Spiritual care of the dying patient. In H. Chochinov & W. Breibart (Eds.), *Handbook of psychiatry in palliative medicine* (pp. 357–373). Oxford Univ. Press.
43. Nelson, C. J., Rosenfeld, B., Breitbart, W., et al. (2002). Spirituality, religion, and depression in the terminally ill. *Psychosomatics, 43*, 213–220.
44. Baider, L., Russak, S. M., Perry, S., et al. (1999). The role of religious and spiritual beliefs in coping with malignant melanoma: An Israeli sample. *Psycho-Oncology, 8*, 417–428.
45. Breitbart, W., & Rosenfeld, B. (1999). Physician-assisted suicide: The influence of psychosocial issues. *Cancer Control, 6*, 146–161.
46. Watson, M., Haviland, J. J., Greer, S., et al. (1999). Influence of psychological response on survival in breast cancer population-based cohort study. *Lancet, 354*, 1331–1336.
47. Rousseau, P. (2000). Spirituality and the dying patient. *Journal of Clinical Oncology, 18*, 2000–2002.
48. Puchalski, C., & Romer, A. L. (2000). Taking a spiritual history allows clinicians to understand patients more fully. *Journal of Palliative Medicine, 3*, 129–137.
49. Post, S. G., Puchalski, C., & Larson, D. B. (2000). Physicians and patient spirituality: Professional boundaries, competency, and ethics. *Annals of Internal Medicine, 132*, 578–583.
50. Gioiella, M. E., Berkman, B., & Robinson, M. (1998). Spirituality and quality of life in gynecologic oncology patients. *Cancer Practice, 6*, 333–338.
51. Schuetz, B. (1995). Spirituality and palliative care. *Australian Family Physician, 24*, 775–777.
52. Bollwinkel, E. M. (1994). Role of spirituality in hospice care. *Annals of the Academy of Medicine, Singapore, 23*, 261–263.
53. Rummans, T. A., Bostwick, J. M., & Clark, M. M. (2000). Mayo Clinic Cancer Center Quality of Life Working Group, Maintaining quality of life at the end of life. *Mayo Clinic Proceedings, 75*, 1305–1310.

54. Koenig, H. G. (2007). Religion and depression in older medical inpatients. *The American Journal of Geriatric Psychiatry, 15*, 282–291.
55. Holland, J. C. (1982). Psychological issues in the care of the terminally ill. In F. Flach F (ed.). *Directions in psychiatry*. Hatherleigh.
56. Lesko, L. M., Massie, M. J., Holland, J. C. (1987). Oncology. In A. Stoudemire & B. S. Fogel (Eds.), *Principles of medical psychiatry*. Grune & Stratton.
57. Heim, E., Augustiny, K. F., Schaffner, L., et al. (1993). Coping with breast cancer over time and situation. *Journal of Psychosomatic Research, 37*, 523–542.
58. Greenstein, M., & Breitbart, W. (2000). Cancer and the experience of meaning: A group psychotherapy program for people with cancer. *American Journal of Psychotherapy, 54*, 486–500.
59. Frankl, V. F. (1955/1986). *The doctor and the soul*. Random House.
60. Frankl, V. F. (1959/1992). *Men's search for meaning* (4th ed.). Beacon Press.
61. Frankl, V. F. (1969/1988). The will to meaning. *Foundations and applications of logotherapy*. Expanded edition. Penguin.
62. Frankl, V. F. (1975/1997). *Men's search for ultimate meaning*. Plenum Press.
63. Balboni, T. A., Paulk, M. E., Balboni, M. J., et al. (2010). Provision of spiritual care to patients with advanced cancer: Association with medical care and quality of life near death. *Journal of Clinical Oncology, 28*, 445–452.
64. Cassem, N. H. (1991). The dying patient. In Cassem (ed.). *MGH handbook of general hospital psychiatry*. Mosby Year Book.
65. Neal, C. (1993). *52 ways to reduce stress in your life*. Thomas Nelson Publishers.

Chapter 7
How to Deal with Spiritual Stressors

7.1 How to Be Free from Guilt

Guilt is a feeling of worry that usually arises from self-blame for moral transgressions. Shame refers to the action tendency to hide evidence of one's failure [1]. It is usually based on the belief that one is inferior to others. He/she cannot tolerate looking foolish to others. In essence, guilt concerns actions, whereas shame concerns perceived self (identity) [2].

Unlike shame, a sense of guilt is difficult to hide [1]. If someone feels guilty, they tend to express it verbally. Thus, guilt can be considered an honest feeling.

If you do not express guilt, your suffering will persist. However, if you express it, the extent of your suffering will be reduced. The problem is that guilt can be sufficiently severe to interfere with daily life.

Many people are afflicted with guilt related to previous wrongdoing. They can feel so for a brief period, but if the guilt is too intense, or if they experience such a feeling repetitively, they are vulnerable to poor health. A sense of guilt can weaken immunity and lead to diseases. These feelings can also cause depression, resulting in suicide [3, 4].

A Vietnam War veteran in his late 40 s was afflicted with feelings of guilt about killing enemies during the war. He consumed alcohol to forget such unpleasant memories. Ultimately, he committed suicide by hanging himself.

Feelings of guilt are not always negative but rather play a positive role by not hurting others. For example, someone who used to abuse children or employees verbally or physically felt guilt toward them and then discontinued the abuse. However, shame can lead to avoidance [5].

People experiencing guilt tend to attribute their present conflict to previous failures. Obsessed with them, they are poor at adapting to their marital and social lives. In such cases, guilt is an escape from reality.

The feeling of guilt is a warning signal that requires one to take measures, such as pain. There are some tips to address guilt [6].

K. B. Koh, *Body, Mind and Spirituality*, https://doi.org/10.1007/978-3-032-11214-9_7

First, make amends when possible.

Someone was afflicted with feelings of guilt because he secretly got on the train many times without paying during his young adulthood. Ten years later, he was free of guilt after paying the train fares to the National Railroad Administration.

If you feel guilty about returning home late at night every day, make it up to your wife by calling her frequently and eating out or taking a trip with her.

Second, recognize your limit.

We must recognize that we are imperfect beings. We are not perfect enough to control everything ourselves. Thus, to describe the limit of human nature, the phrase "To err is human, to forgive is divine" was coined by the English poet Alexander Pope. We must remember that we can learn and grow through mistakes and failures.

Third, be more faithful to your work to drive out the ghost of your past.

If you focus on work that can satisfy you, you will be free from your preoccupation with past events. A woman in her 30 s felt guilty about having sex with her ex-lover after her engagement to another man and was depressed. Learning embroidery and teaching English, she was free from her sense of guilt and overcame depression.

Finally, talk to another person about your guilty feelings, if possible.

A married woman was afflicted with a sense of guilt about having sex with another man before her marriage. She was anxious, irritable, and unable to sleep well, saying, "I am an unforgivable woman."

Unable to withstand her suffering, she visited the department of psychiatry of a general hospital to consult a psychiatrist. She was free from guilt after talking to a psychiatrist several times.

It is important to express one's hidden feelings toward someone. Guilt grows secretly. The more you hide it, the greater your feelings of guilt. Ultimately, you are likely to become psychologically and physically ill.

However, if you are concerned about talking to another person who may add to your guilt, it might be more helpful to see a professional consultant, including a psychiatrist, rather than talking to people around you.

If you cannot talk anywhere, confess to God: "Pour out your hearts to him, for God is our refuge (Psalms 62:8)."

7.2 How to Forgive

If you learn to forgive others, your life becomes qualitatively different. Otherwise, you will bear a grudge against them, triggering you to harm them and yourself.

Some people say, "I won't forgive him at all until I die." Holding such a deep grudge and anger can hurt your health more than others. These individuals are likely to have cancer or coronary heart disease, as well as depression [7–12].

One day, Leonardo da Vinci became very angry at someone while painting "The Last Supper." He cried and hurled abuses at him. After that, he gripped the brush again to paint the picture, but could not because angry Jesus came to his mind. He was angry at himself.

He stopped painting the picture, went to the person who had made him angry, and sought forgiveness. After receiving forgiveness, he could complete painting Jesus' face.

One woman with breast cancer showed strong resentment and hostility toward her husband, who had shown little concern about her situation. After reading the part "Forgive" in the book "Anger Kills," she began to change her attitude and forgive her husband, followed by lessening hostility and its consequent symptoms, such as seething.

Nelson Mandela was in prison for a long time and was tortured after being arrested while fighting racial discrimination in South Africa. However, after becoming the president of the country, he chose reconciliation instead of revenge against white people. His forgiveness prevented the country from falling into unhappiness.

Although it is difficult to forgive others, peace cannot be achieved without forgiveness. Ultimately, we must choose between war and forgiveness.

The following Bible verse informs us of what to do when we have an unforgivable person:

> "Love your enemies, do good to them, and lend to them without expecting to get anything back. Then your reward will be great (Luke 6:35)."

If it is hard for you to forgive someone, pray for him: "Let me have compassion to forgive him."

7.3 Prayer

Prayers can calm you. Let us pray before going to bed, close your eyes, and look back at the day. I would like you to give thanks for this day and ask for wisdom on things to do in the future. You can see the next day anew with peace of mind. Prayers can help you maintain spiritual health.

Prayers can also help manage stress in many ways [13]. Only bowing your head and closing your eyes for prayer at regular times during the day will provide you with relief. Prayer can be a time of personal reflection that changes one's attitude and perspective to cope well with stress.

Praying for others [14, 15] is a source of social support [16]. For those suffering from illness or facing difficulties in life, prayer can help them cope well or recover quickly by getting together with others who encourage them, not by themselves.

Here are some tips on how to pray to relieve stress [13].

7.3.1 Pray Regularly

Pray regularly, rather than just when under extreme stress. By making prayers a regular practice, you will enjoy the ongoing benefits of meditation and personal reflection, and you will develop a close relationship with God. When you have a familiar relationship with God, you will have more faith that God is hearing your prayers and will respond when you are stressed.

7.3.2 Give Thanks

When you pray, express thanks to God for the good things in your life. Counting your blessings in prayer can put life stressors into perspective, so that they are less overwhelming.

7.3.3 Ask for Wisdom

Ask God for wisdom. Sometimes, life gets out of control, and you cannot figure out how to change your life to reduce stress. At such times, ask God for wisdom to reduce stress or manage the stress that you cannot escape.

7.3.4 Confess

Tell God about things you have done that you regret and you will feel relieved. In the end, it will be possible to free you from the stress caused by your guilt.

7.3.5 Hand Over Your Worries

The Bible says, "Cast all your anxiety upon him because he cares for you" (1 Peter 5:7). When you pray, take all your anxiety and worries to God. Ask God to take care of them. When these anxieties and worries begin to weigh on you again, remind yourself that they are in God's capable hands.

7.3.6 Ask What You Want

Ask God to reveal anything about your attitude or actions that you need to change. Believe that God is listening to and will answer your prayers. There will be times when you must ask your Father for something. Just because you do not always get what you seek, do not stop praying. God may withhold things he knows will not be good for you in the long run. In this case, one must wait until God's timing makes it obvious.

7.3.7 Request Specifically

Pray as specifically as possible. For example, instead of praying, "God, bless my friend," pray, "God, please help my friend find a job."

7.3.8 How to Pray: ACTS

ACTS is an acronym for the prayer method that involves adoration, confession, thanksgiving, and supplication. It is a simple, four-step way of praying to help connect with God.

What each step of the ACTS prayer method means:

Adoration: Expressing praise and worship for God.

Confession: Acknowledging your sins and asking for forgiveness

Thanksgiving: Giving thanks for what God has done for you.

Supplication: Asking God for what you need, such as help with a problem or guidance on a decision.

This acronym can serve as a guide, especially when learning how to pray.

If you are unfamiliar with prayers, recite a written prayer every night or morning. It will then be able to help bring about serenity.

7.4 Pretend Today Is Your Last

We live with the thought that we will live tomorrow like we lived yesterday. Therefore, we cannot forgive someone who broke our heart and then spend our day holding a grudge against them. However, if you consider today as your last day, you can forgive them.

Pretend that you have just heard from your doctor the terrible news that you have a fatal illness and have only a few weeks to live. Even though you have made a great fortune, what will it mean to you? Moreover, if today is the only day you can live on earth, will you have anyone you cannot forgive?

Patients who had a heart attack tended to walk away from anger, although they used to be angry before the attack [17].

Are you facing a difficult situation? Do you have anyone you cannot forgive now? If you say, "Yes," pretend "today is your last day." It will orient you toward thinking differently about any difficult things or unforgivable person, saying, "That's not great."

Sometimes, such thoughts give you room to think positively and change your life qualitatively.

7.5 Love Can Work a Miracle [6]

I was impressed by the movie "The Miracle Worker" a long time ago. It was about Helen Keller, who was born blind, deaf, and mute, and finally grew up as a great person who served disabled people.

Ms. Sullivan's love made Keller great. This achievement was the result of her love. She taught and disciplined the hopeless and uncontrollable Helen Keller with love and perseverance.

Many people around us did not receive love and suffered from either depression or physical suffering. In other words, the lack of love makes one not only depressed, but it also hurts them physically.

In recent years, a growing number of people engage in doctor shopping because of their pain but do not experience any improvement. They finally visit the department of psychiatry.

A man in his mid-40 s underwent various laboratory examinations and received treatment for backache at the department of orthopedic surgery. However, the patient showed no improvement with painkillers. His pain was so severe that he could not use the toilet. Therefore, his wife had to help him urinate using a bucket.

He felt there was not much to live for because of marital conflict and his wife's refusal to have sex with him, and his being unwillingly transferred to another place. In this situation, the backache recurred. The pain was too severe to tolerate, unlike the previous pain.

Surprisingly, an unusual event occurred. His wife, who refused to have sex due to feeling tired, looked quite different after he began to suffer from a backache. She willingly helped him urinate, traveled far, and returned several times a day to help him with his illness. He said to himself, "How could she do that?" "If I were in her shoes, could I do that?".

He once thought about divorce because of his wife's cold attitude and indifference. However, his attitude toward his wife changed after seeing her devotion to him: "No woman better than my wife!" "I will be better to her if I get well."

He felt ashamed of his narrow-minded attitude toward his wife. He also began to recognize the true meaning of life and expressed confidence about creating a new life. With this thought, his backache dramatically improved even without taking painkillers.

His backache recurred because he was dissatisfied with his wife, and then improved because of her devotion to him. Not only did his backache improve, but the window of his narrow mind also widened.

His view of the world changed. As seen in him, love has the magical power to change a person.

7.6 Summary

1. This chapter dealt with not only spiritual stressors, such as guilt and forgiveness, but also how to be free from guilt and how to forgive.
2. "Pretend today is your last" will help orient you toward thinking differently about any difficult things or unforgivable people.
3. Some tips on how to pray to relieve stress were mentioned.
4. As seen in a clinical case, love has the magical power to change a person.

References

1. Lazarus, R. S. (1993). Why we should think of stress as a subset of emotion. In L. Goldberger & S. Breznitz (Eds.), *Handbook of stress: Theoretical and clinical aspects* (2nd ed.). The Free Press.
2. Tracy, J. L., & Robins, R. W. (2006). Appraisal antecedents of shame and guilt: Support for a theoretical model. *Personality and Social Psychology Bulletin, 32*, 1339–1351.
3. Breslau, N., & Davis, C. D. (1985). Refining DSM-III criteria in major depression: An assessment of the descriptive validity of criterion symptoms. *Journal of Affective Disorders, 9*, 199–206.
4. Jarrett, R. B., & Weissenberger, J. E. (1990). Guilt in depressed outpatients. *Journal of Consulting and Clinical Psychology, 58*, 495–498.
5. Tangney, J. P., & Dearing, R. (2002). *Shame and guilt in interpersonal relationships.* Guilford Press.
6. Koh, K. B. (1999). *Ways to keep myself from all kinds of stressors.* Haneon.
7. Hecker, M. H. L., Chesney, M. A., Black, G. W., et al. (1988). Coronary-prone behaviors in the western collaborative group study. *Psychosomatic Medicine, 50*, 153–164.
8. Koh, K. B., Cho, S. Y., Kim, J. W., et al. (2004). The relationship of anger expression and alexithymia with coronary artery stenosis in patients with coronary artery diseases. *Yonsei Medical Journal, 45*, 181–186.
9. Koh, K. B. (2018). *Stress and Somatic Symptoms: Biopsychosociospiritual Perspectives.* Springer.
10. Siegman, A. W., Dembroski, T. M., & Ringel, N. (1987). Components of hostility and severity of coronary artery disease. *Psychosomatic Medicine, 49*, 127–135.
11. Greer, S., & Morris, T. (1975). Psychological attributes of women who develop breast cancer: A controlled study. *Journal of Psychosomatic Research, 19*, 147–153.
12. Abse, D. W., Wilkins, M. M., & Van de Castle, R. L. (1974). Personality and behavioral characteristics of lung cancer patients. *Journal of Psychosomatic Research, 18*, 101–113.
13. Neal, C. (1993). *52 ways to reduce stress in your life.* Thomas Nelson Publishers.
14. Taylor, R. J., & Chatters, L. M. (1988). Church members as a source of informal social support. *Review of Religious Research, 30*, 193–202.
15. Maton, K. I. (1989). Community settings as buffers of life stress? Highly supportive churches, mutual help groups, and senior centers. *American Journal of Community Psychology, 17*, 203–232.
16. Sullivan, W. P. (1993). It helps me to be a whole person: The role of spirituality among the mentally challenged. *Psychosocial Rehabilitation Journal, 16*, 125–134.
17. Williams, R., & Williams, V. (1993). *Anger kills: Seventeen strategies for controlling the hostility that can harm your health.* Times Books.

Part III
Resilience-Enhancing Approaches to Somatization

Chapter 8
Interview Techniques for Managing Somatizing Patients

8.1 What Is Somatization?

Somatization is a process in which there is an inappropriate focus on physical symptoms while denying psychosocial problems [1]. Patients with somatic symptom and related disorders (SSRDs) are more likely to overinterpret and catastrophize physical symptoms than patients with depressive or anxiety disorders [2].

Somatization is highly prevalent in primary care where 20%–30% of patients fulfill the criteria for SSRDs (DSM-5) [3–5].

Despite its high prevalence, somatization often goes unrecognized [4, 6]. Patients with SSRDs are called "medical orphans" [7] because they doctor shop but cannot find a willing physician. They suffer from long-term distress and seek treatment, which often results in disappointment because the correct diagnosis is not made by physicians. They often complain that their symptoms are genuine, but their medical tests generally yield negative results [8].

8.2 Rationale for Using a Special Interview Technique in Somatizing Patients

The treatment of SSRDs is challenging because they cannot be treated according to the existing biomedical model and patients with SSRDs are usually resistant to a psychosocial approach [9]. Physicians may be less skilled in providing support and care in a background of diagnostic uncertainty [10]. Moreover, somatic symptoms persist despite treatment [8], leaving patients dissatisfied with their management. This may be because clinicians do not effectively address patients' needs beyond the management of pathology [11].

Research on primary and secondary care in the United Kingdom has shown that patients primarily expect explanations and understanding, which are more important

K. B. Koh, *Body, Mind and Spirituality*, https://doi.org/10.1007/978-3-032-11214-9_8

than expectations for support, testing, and diagnosis [12, 13]. Therefore, specific assessment skills and treatment techniques are required to effectively treat patients with SSRDs, for whom the acceptance of psychiatric treatment is essential [1].

8.3 Interview Techniques for Physicians

Physicians must learn some important interview techniques for the effective assessment and management of SSRDs.

8.3.1 Empathetic Listening and Patience

Empathetic listening is critical to effective patient-centered care [8]. Management of patients with SSRDs often requires patience from physicians because patients may be angry and dissatisfied, feeling that they are not being taken seriously [11]. At the same time, some physicians cannot tolerate patients' frequent complaints and demands, showing anger toward such patients not only because their illness behavior is different from other patients' but also because their symptoms are not medically explained. This countertransference can be frequently observed during the management of patients with SSRDs [14, 15], which leads to the disruption of the doctor-patient relationship.

8.3.2 Accept the Patient's Suffering

People who suffer from an undiagnosed illness want their symptoms to be acknowledged as "genuine." They also want to be assured that practitioners will work with them to suggest and negotiate strategies that may help alleviate their symptoms and better "manage" their situation. Therefore, physicians should accept such patients' suffering as legitimate. In addition, physicians should avoid a strict mind–body dualism when explaining symptoms [8].

8.3.3 Biopsychosocial Assessment

There is no dichotomy between physical and psychological disorders. Rather, the proportion of physical or psychological etiology varies across a continuum [16]. Psychological factors such as health anxiety and symptom attributions may influence the genesis and presentation of physical symptoms, even in the absence of psychiatric disorders. Therefore, from the beginning of assessment, equal attention should be devoted to understanding biopsychosocial factors, such as somatic, psychological, and environmental aspects in patients with SSRDs [11]. When taking the patient's history, physicians should be aware of psychosocial cues and then should be consistent and unambiguous in their management of the patients [1].

Understand the Patient's Illness Experience

Physicians must understand the problems faced by patients with SSRDs. One way to help these patients is for physicians to adopt patient-centered care. Physicians trained in biomedical models of care may be able to satisfactorily identify and treat diseases but be less at ease in providing care and support. By contrast, patient-centered care, with its emphasis on not only the disease but also the illness experience, may provide a framework for physicians to provide enhanced care and support [17].

Patient-centered care also stresses the importance of finding common ground with the patient. In relation to SSRDs, it may be particularly helpful for physicians and patients to reach a mutual understanding and agreement of the problems. If a full biomedical explanation is not possible, then partial explanations that are consistent with the patient's point of view may be valuable to patients' outcomes [18].

Learn Communication Skills

Once patients with SSRDs have been identified by physicians, these physicians need to develop the following skills:

(1) Let the patient know his/her potential diagnosis and its prognosis by explaining test results and the nature of the illness.
(2) Use general terms such as "tension" and "stress" and avoid using professional (or psychological) terms to minimize patients' resistance [9].
(3) Explain the mechanisms of somatization by giving an example of common somatic symptoms, such as palpitation, headache, and backache [1, 19].
(4) Make sure patients will improve when they receive treatment from specialists, such as psychiatrists.
(5) Administer the appropriate treatment, which may or may not involve psychiatric referral [1].

How to Refer the Patient for Psychiatric or Psychological Assessment

Physicians should learn how to refer patients with SSRDs for psychiatric or psychological assessment [1] because these patients show resistance to psychological explanations [8]. First, physicians should inform patients about their negative test results and provide explanations for the symptoms [1]. Second, medical students and physicians should be trained to give the patient positive messages based on positive experiences of the therapeutic process for patients with SSRDs during their clinical clerkship and based on physicians' clinical experiences. For example, such statements may include "I've seen many patients get better after they were referred to specialists and received treatment." Finally, they should develop their skills for referral by practicing this experience or using role-playing.

The above-mentioned effective approach to patients with SSRDs for physicians is presented in the Fig. 8.1 [20].

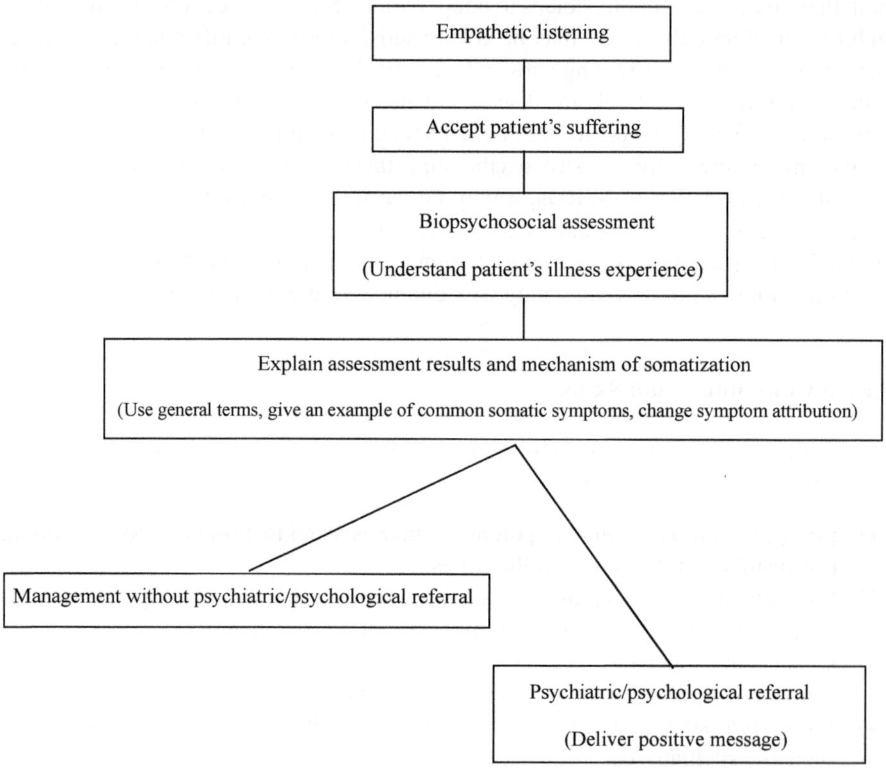

Fig. 8.1 An effective approach to somatization assessment and management for physicians (From Koh [20])

8.4 Education for Medical Students and Primary Care Physicians

Patients with SSRDs are good candidates for medical students and primary care physicians to learn about the biopsychosocial approach for patient-centered care because their symptoms cannot be biomedically explained. Primary care physicians also feel that effective management strategies are lacking [21, 22]. Therefore, psychological skills should be taught to medical students during their clinical rotations and general practitioners during their training period. During these training periods, psychiatrists play an important role in helping other physicians develop the skills necessary to identify and manage patients with SSRDs [1].

Educational programs should include information about somatization such as the diagnostic criteria for SSRDs [23]; the role of stress, anger, and mood in these disorders [1, 24]; skills training in biopsychosocial history taking; a general treatment model for SSRDs; and advice on the management of chronic cases [23].

8.5 Summary

1. Patients with SSRDs require explanations and understanding from physicians beyond their expectations for support, testing, and diagnosis. However, non-psychiatric physicians should avoid mind–body dualism.
2. From the beginning of the assessment, equal attention should be devoted to each biopsychosocial factor affecting patients with SSRDs. In particular, physicians need to adopt patient-centered care with its emphasis not only on the disease but also on the illness experience as a way of helping these patients.
3. Medical students and primary physicians should learn how to refer patients with SSRDs for psychiatric and psychological assessments. Role-playing is effective in teaching psychological skills (e.g., interview techniques) to medical students and general practitioners.
4. A positive explanation for the possible causes of the disease, combined with an optimistic prognosis, may be effective for the management and referral of patients with SSRDs.

References

1. Bass, C., & Benjamin, S. (1993). The management of chronic somatization. *British Journal of Psychiatry, 162*, 472–480.
2. Rief, W., Hiller, W., & Margraf, J. (1998). Cognitive aspects of hypochondriasis and the somatization syndrome. *Journal of Abnormal Psychology, 107*, 587–595.

3. Toft, T., Fink, P., & Oernboel, E., et al. (2005). Mental disorders in primary care: prevalence and co-morbidity among disorders. Results from the functional illness in primary care (FIP) study. *Psychological Medicine, 35*, 1175–1184.
4. Fink, P., Sorensen, L., & Engberg, M., et al. (1999). Somatization in primary care. Prevalence, health care utilization, and general practitioner recognition. *Psychosomatics, 40*, 330–338.
5. Arnold, I. A., de Waal, M. W., Eekhof, J. A., et al. (2006). Somatoform disorder in primary care: Course and the need for cognitive-behavioral treatment. *Psychosomatics, 47*, 498–503.
6. Goldberg, D., & Bridges, K. (1987). Screening for psychiatric illness in general practice: The general practitioner versus the screening questionnaire. *The Journal of the Royal College of General Practitioners, 37*, 15–18.
7. Aronowitz, R. A. (2001). When do symptoms become a disease? *Annals of Internal Medicine, 134*, 803–808.
8. Nettleton, S., Watt, I., O'Malley, L., et al. (2005). Understanding the narratives of people who live with medically unexplained illness. *Patient Education and Counseling, 56*, 205–210.
9. Koh, K. B. (2011). Stress and psychosomatic medicine. *Seoul: Ilchokak*, 263–285.
10. Rhodes, L. A., McPhillips-Tangum, C. A., Markham, C., et al. (1999). The power of the visible: The meaning of diagnostic tests in chronic back pain. *Social Science and Medicine, 48*, 1189–1203.
11. Price, J. R. (2000). Managing physical symptoms: The clinical assessment as treatment. *Journal of Psychosomatic Research, 48*, 1–10.
12. Williams, S., Weinman, J., Dale, J., et al. (1995). Patient expectations: What do primary care patients want from the GP and how far does meeting expectations affect patient satisfaction? *Family Practice, 12*, 193–201.
13. Matthews, D. A., Sledge, W. H., Lieberman, P. B., et al. (1987). Evaluation of intern performance by medical inpatients. *American Journal of Medicine, 35*, 936–944.
14. Gorlin, R., & Zucker, H. D. (1983). Physician's reactions to patients: A key to teaching humanistic medicine. *New England Journal of Medicine, 308*, 1059–1063.
15. Groves, J. E. (1978). Taking care of the hateful patient. *New England Journal of Medicine, 298*, 883–887.
16. Mayou, R. A., Bass, C., & Sharpe, M. (1995). *Treatment of functional somatic symptoms*. Oxford University Press.
17. Stewart, M., Brown, J., Weston, W., et al. (2003). *Patient-centered medicine transforming the clinical method*. Radcliffe Medical Press.
18. Salmon, P. (2000). Patients who present with physical symptoms in the absence of physical pathology: A challenge to existing models of doctor-patient interaction. *Patient Education and Counseling, 39*, 105–113.
19. Sharpe, M., & Bass, C. (1992). Pathophysiological mechanisms in somatization. *International Review of Psychiatry, 4*, 81–97.
20. Koh, K. B. (2013). An effective approach to somatization assessment and management. In K. B. Koh (Ed.), *Somatization and psychosomatic symptoms* (pp. 99–111). Springer.
21. Kerwick, S., Jones, R., Mann, A., et al. (1997). Mental health care training priorities in general practice. *British Journal of General Practice, 47*, 225–227.
22. Reid, S., Whooley, D., Crayford, T., et al. (2001). Medically unexplained symptoms – GPs' attitudes towards their cause and management. *Family Practice, 18*, 519–523.
23. Fink, P., Rosendal, M., & Toft, T. (2002). Assessment and treatment of functional disorders in general practice: The extended reattribution and management model – An advanced educational program for nonpsychiatric doctors. *Psychosomatics, 43*, 93–131.
24. Koh, K. B., Kim, D. K., Kim, S. Y., et al. (2008). The relation between anger management style, mood, and somatic symptoms in anxiety disorders and somatoform disorders. *Psychiatry Research, 160*, 372–379.

Chapter 9
General Management of Somatic Symptom and Related Disorders

9.1 The Basic Premise of Psychological Interventions in Somatization

1. Somatization is a universal phenomenon and often a direct consequence of common emotional symptoms, such as anxiety or depression (i.e., autonomic arousal symptoms or somatic complaints) [1].
2. The perception, appraisal, and interpretation of the bodily sensations are known to be influenced by personal factors such as cognitions about health [2].
3. The following cognitive consequences of symptoms contribute to the maintenance of these symptoms:

(a) Selective attention increases worry and heightens awareness of physical symptoms.

(b) Catastrophic thinking about the potentially harmful origin of bodily sensations results in fear, additional symptoms, or a lower threshold for symptom perception [3].

9.2 Psychological Interventions

Psychological interventions in somatization can be broadly classified into referral by physicians and management by trained physicians or psychiatrists using cognitive behavioral techniques [3].

However, an overemphasis on the psychosocial causation of somatic symptoms may further alienate these patients. Biologically unexplained somatic symptoms are not only a source of distress and dissatisfaction for patients but also pose a challenge for healthcare professionals. Unfortunately, these concerns are often neglected by psychiatrists [4–7].

K. B. Koh, *Body, Mind and Spirituality*, https://doi.org/10.1007/978-3-032-11214-9_9

Sharpe et al. [2] proposed a biopsychosocial model to understand unexplained physical symptoms, which takes all the biopsychosocial aspects into consideration. In this context, cognitive behavioral techniques are considered crucial for the assessment and management of patients with such symptoms. Additionally, psychiatric consultations and psychopharmacological treatment can be employed.

9.3 Cognitive Behavioral Therapy

Cognitive behavioral therapy (CBT) has been shown to be effective for patients with somatic symptom and related disorders (SSRDs) [8]. The central idea of this approach is to focus on the consequences rather than the causes of symptoms, providing an opportunity to treat physical symptoms without fruitless discussion of causes. This approach considers the interactions of biopsychosocial factors in the perception and maintenance of somatic symptoms [2].

CBT components are as follows [3]:

1. Relaxation techniques to reduce physiological arousal
2. Engagement in pleasurable and meaningful activities to reduce strain or prevent overwork
3. Linking emotions and the intensity of symptoms
4. Modification of dysfunctional beliefs through cognitive restructuring
5. Behavioral experiments to challenge the symptom-related catastrophic beliefs
6. Reducing reinforcement of illness behavior

Other components include problem-solving training, assertiveness training, visualization, graded increases in activity level, coping skills training, exercise, and breathing training [3].

9.3.1 Cognitive Therapy in Medical Care

Cognitive factors may contribute to the genesis of all physical symptoms and the associated distress, disability, and healthcare use. Physical symptoms have two essential components: awareness of bodily sensations and attribution of abnormalities to the sensation. In particular, attributions influence a sufferer's response to sensations. Therefore, cognitions such as symptom attributions clearly play a role in the presentation of physical symptoms in medical care [9].

Cognitive therapy is a psychological treatment that aims to alter symptom attributions, thereby improving outcomes in the treatment of persistent and troubling physical symptoms.

This therapy is usually conducted individually in ten or more weekly sessions of approximately 1 h each. Patients are actively involved in testing and modifying their dysfunctional beliefs regarding their physical symptoms. However, cognitive therapy is time-consuming and expensive [9].

The two obstacles to the availability and acceptability of cognitive therapy can be overcome by integrating aspects of cognitive therapy into medical care [9]. Cognitive therapy for medically unexplained physical symptoms and hypochondriasis includes identifying and challenging patients' evidence of misinterpretation of bodily sensations [2, 10]. In a general hospital clinic, the clinician may act as a cognitive therapist by eliciting the patient's beliefs, explaining their view about the cause of the symptoms, presenting evidence from the assessment to support their view, and, if appropriate, challenging the patient's view. Therefore, clinical assessments such as history taking, physical examination, and testing may modify cognitive factors such as symptom attribution and consequently improve outcomes [9]. These findings may provide evidence that can be used to confirm or refute patients' beliefs. If symptoms remain medically unexplained, a positive explanation of the possible causes combined with an optimistic prognosis may be effective [9].

However, formal cognitive therapy cannot be offered to every patient presenting with physical symptoms, because such an approach would not be acceptable to many patients.

9.3.2 Mindfulness-Based Cognitive Therapy

Mindfulness-Based Cognitive Therapy (MBCT) is a psychological therapy designed to prevent the relapse of depression [11]. It uses a combination of CBT methods and psychological strategies such as mindfulness and mindfulness meditation.

The goal of the MBCT is to interrupt recurring automatic cognitive processes and teach participants to focus less on reacting to incoming stimuli and instead accept and observe them without judgment [12].

MBCT can help improve mental functioning (e.g., vitality and social functioning) in patients with persistent and medically unexplained symptoms, although it may not improve physical functioning [13]. Changes in unhealthy behavioral patterns and increased self-care and self-compassion can also result from this process [14]. In particular, the increase in use of mental health care after MBCT indicated that patients with SSRDs became more willing to engage in mental health care. This highlights MBCT as a potentially meaningful intervention for this population [15].

9.4 Psychiatric Consultation as a Therapeutic Strategy

Psychiatric consultation is one of the most effective interventions for patients with SSRDs, as defined by the DSM-5 [16]. Psychiatric consultation followed by a management planning letter offers only modest benefits in terms of health status and patient satisfaction [17]. At that time, psychiatric consultation could be effectively used as a moderator in the transition from primary physicians to psychiatrists to minimize patients' resistance to the direct psychiatric approach [18].

9.5 Psychopharmacotherapy

Psychopharmacotherapy is essential for the management of patients with SSRDs for several reasons [19]:

1. A high proportion of patients with SSRDs have comorbid anxiety and depressive disorders, which are often underdetected and inadequately treated. Occasionally, somatic presentations may reflect an underlying depressive or anxiety disorder.
2. Medications are more acceptable to patients as they may feel relieved to learn that something is wrong and treatment is available.
3. Pharmacotherapy is relatively cost-effective, simple, and straightforward.
4. Physicians are more at ease in prescribing medication rather than exploring psychosocial causes of somatic symptoms, which are often speculative and lack definitive proof.
5. Selective serotonin reuptake inhibitors (SSRIs) and serotonin and noradrenaline reuptake inhibitors (SNRIs) act both peripherally and centrally to reduce the perception of pain and other heightened perceptions, which are common presenting symptoms in patients with SSRDs [20, 21]. Common side effects of some antidepressants, such as somnolence and increased appetite, can be a therapeutic advantage, especially for patients with poor sleep and appetite.

In clinical practice, all classes of psychotropics, such as tricyclic antidepressants, SSRIs, SNRIs, antianxiety agents, atypical antipsychotics, and herbal medications, are effective in a wide range of disorders. Particularly, antidepressants appear to be effective against SSRDs [19].

9.5.1 Antidepressants

Antidepressants are the most commonly used drugs for patients with SSRDs. There is merit in using antidepressants for several reasons: pain is often a common presenting symptom in patients with somatic symptom disorder, and antidepressants have analgesic properties. Additionally, somatic symptoms may present as undiagnosed anxiety or depressive disorder [20–22].

Antidepressants with the dual action of serotonin and noradrenaline, such as SNRIs (e.g., venlafaxine and duloxetine), seem more effective than other antidepressants if pain is the main symptom, whereas SSRIs (e.g., fluoxetine and paroxetine) seem to be more effective in treating illness anxiety disorder (formerly hypochondriasis) [19].

The dosages and main side effects of the antidepressants used in adults and older patients are described in Chap. 12 (Table 12.1). In general, it is safe to start one-third of the usual adult dosage of antidepressants in older patients [23].

To prevent side effects, such as anxiety, restlessness, and recurrence of depression, antidepressant medications should not be discontinued abruptly under any circumstances. Medications need to be tapered slowly over a 1- to 2-week period [24, 25].

Sexual dysfunction and weight gain may become apparent within one month of starting an SSRI. However, it should be noted that more than 50% of patients with major depressive disorder may have sexual dysfunction as a symptom of their depression [26]. Among antidepressants, SSRIs and venlafaxine are more likely to cause sexual dysfunction than duloxetine and bupropion [27].

The following treatment options are available for patients whose depression has improved while taking an antidepressant, but in whom sexual dysfunction develops during therapy [24]: (1) reduce the dose of the antidepressant, (2) take a drug holiday, and (3) switch medications (e.g., duloxetine or bupropion).

Moreover, weight gain may occur with the use of antidepressants in patients with diabetes [24]. In particular, tricyclic antidepressants such as amitriptyline and SSRIs such as paroxetine can cause weight gain. Fluoxetine may cause weight loss when used for less than 6 months and weight gain when used for more than 6 months [28].

To manage weight gain associated with antidepressant treatment, patients are recommended to improve their diet and initiate exercise programs, and the medication should be changed to weight-neutral medications (e.g., duloxetine and bupropion).

9.5.2 Practical Issues for Psychopharmacotherapy

The following factors are important in planning psychopharmacological treatment for patients with SSRDs [19].

1. Provide symptomatic treatment until a definite etiology and intervention are identified.
2. Prepare patients for psychopharmacotherapy by explaining the rationale, expected outcomes, and common adverse effects before initiation of medication.
3. Focus on care rather than cause or cure.
4. Aim to improve quality of life.
5. Focus on relief, coping, and return to function.
6. Provide adequate trials for at least 12 weeks before declaring any drug ineffective and explaining it to patients so that they can expect improvement over several weeks or months.
7. Emphasize that different treatments may act synergistically. Psychological treatments are not substitutes for pharmacological treatment; different treatments are complementary.

8. Start at a low dose and titrate gradually over weeks, as these patients are usually sensitive to side effects. Compliance can be an issue if the medication is titrated too quickly.

9.6 Integrated Therapy

Considering the time limitations for physicians, an integrated brief therapy is recommended for patients with SSRDs. This form of therapy should be multimodal, combining the effective components of therapies from different therapeutic models [3]. In particular, integrating psychiatric consultation, CBT, and psychopharmacological treatment is considered beneficial.

9.7 Primary Care Treatment for Somatization

Primary care treatment for SSRDs generally follows two main approaches. One approach is shared care, in which mental health specialists offer patient assessment and treatment guidelines [29]. Another approach involves educating primary care physicians to improve their management of somatization within their own settings using the reattribution model [29, 30].

Research [31] suggests that physicians may benefit from long-term training from specialists, such as psychiatrists, to more effectively manage patients with SSRDs. Otherwise, physicians should focus on the referral process rather than on management.

9.8 Summary

1. Cognitive behavioral therapy (CBT) is known to be effective in patients with somatic symptoms and related disorders (SSRDs).
2. History taking, physical examination, and investigations can be used to confirm or refute the patients' beliefs.
3. Mindfulness-based cognitive therapy (MBCT) can be considered a meaningful therapy for patients with SSRDs because it encourages them to be more willing to receive mental healthcare.
4. Psychiatric consultation can be used as a therapeutic strategy. Additionally, psychopharmacotherapy is essential for the management of somatization.
5. Considering the time limitations for physicians, integrated brief therapy is recommended for such patients. This form of therapy should be multimodal, combining psychiatric consultation, CBT, and psychopharmacotherapy.

The Author's Message

Whenever I encounter patients with somatic symptom disorder, I believe their personal needs and views of illness should be understood and respected. On one hand, managing such patients requires empathetic patience from therapists. On the other hand, love and care from an important person involved in their conflict may serve as a panacea for their illness in some cases.

References

1. Patel, V., & Sumathipala, A. (2006). Psychological approaches to somatization in developing countries. *Advances in Pychiatr Treatments, 12*, 54–62.
2. Sharpe, M., Peveler, R., & Mayou, R. (1992). The psychological treatment of patients with functional somatic symptoms: A practical guide. *Journal of Psychosomatic Research, 36*, 515–529.
3. Sharma, M. P., & Manjula, M. (2013). Behavioral and psychological management of somatic symptom disorders: An overview. *International Review of Psychiatry, 25*, 116–124.
4. Bass, C., & Benjamin, S. (1993). The management of chronic somatization. *British Journal of Psychiatry, 162*, 472–480.
5. Bass, C., Peveler, R., & House, A. (2001). Somatoform disorder: Severe psychiatric illnesses neglected by psychiatrists. *British Journal of Psychiatry, 179*, 11–14.
6. Fink, P., & Rosenthal, M. (2008). Recent developments in the understanding and management of functional somatic symptoms in primary care. *Current Opinion in Psychiatry, 21*, 182–188.
7. Kroenke, K. (2003). Patients presenting with somatic complaints: Epidemiology, psychiatric comorbidity and management. *International Journal of Methods in Psychiatric Research, 12*, 34–43.
8. Kroenke, K. (2007). Efficacy of treatment for somatoform disorders: A review of randomized controlled trials. *Psychosomatic Medicine, 69*, 881–888.
9. Price, J. R. (2000). Managing physical symptoms: The clinical assessment as treatment. *Journal of Psychosomatic Research, 48*, 1–10.
10. Salkovskis, P. M. (1989). Somatic problems. In K. Hawton, P. M. Salkovskis, J. Kirk et al. (Eds.), *Cogntive behavior therapy for psychiatric problems. A practical guide*. Oxford University Press.
11. Piet, J., & Hougaard, E. (2011). The effect of mindfulness-based cognitive therapy for prevention of relapse in recurrent major depressive disorder: A systematic review and meta-analysis. *Clinical Psychology Review, 31*, 1032–1040.
12. Felder, J. N., Dimidjian, S., & Segal, Z. (2012). Collaboration in Mindfulness-Based Cognitive Therapy. *Journal of Clinical Psychology, 68*, 179–186.
13. van Ravesteijn, H., Lucassen, P., Bor, H., et al. (2013). Mindfulness-based cognitive therapy for patients with medically unexplained symptoms: A randomized controlled trial. *Psychotherapy and Psychosomatics, 82*, 299–310.
14. van Ravesteijn, H., Suijkerbuijk, Y. B., Langbroek, J. A., et al. (2014). Mindfulness-based cognitive therapy for patients with medically unexplained symptoms: Process of change. *Journal of Psychosomatic Research, 77*, 27–33.
15. van Ravesteijn, H. (2016). Mindfulness-based cognitive therapy for patients with somatoform disorders. *Tijdschrift voor Psychiatrie, 58*, 198–206.
16. Smith, G. R., Jr. (1991). Effectiveness of treatment for somatoform disorder patients. *Psychiatric Medication, 9*, 545–558.
17. van der Feltz-Cornelis, C. M., van Oppen, P., Ader, H. J., et al. (2006). Randomized controlled trial of a collaborative care model with psychiatric consultation for persistent medically unexplained symptoms in general practice. *Psychotherapy and Psychosomatics, 75*, 282–289.

18. Strain, J. J. (2000). Consultation-liaison psychiatry. In B. J. Sadock, V. A. Sadock (Eds.), *Comprehensive textbook of psychiatry* (7th ed.). Lippincott Williams & Wilkins.
19. Somashekar, B., Jainer, A., & Wuntakal, B. (2013). Psychopharmacotherapy of somatic symptoms disorders. *International Review of Psychiatry, 25*, 107–115.
20. Linch, M. E. (2001). Antidepressants as analgesics: A review of randomized controlled trials. *Journal of Psychiatry & Neuroscience, 26*, 30–36.
21. Sussman, N. (2003). SNRIs versus SSRIs: Mechanisms of action in treating depressions and painful physical symptoms. *Primary Care Companion Journal of Clinical Psychiatry, 5*, 19–26.
22. Fishbain, D. A., Cutler, R. B., & Rosomoff, H. L. (1998). Do antidepressants have an analgesic effect in psychogenic pain and somatoform pain disorder? *A meta-analysis. Psychosomatic Medicine, 60*, 503–509.
23. Min, S. K. (2006). *New Psychiatry*. Ilchokak.
24. Unger, J., & Schwartz, Z. (2013). *Diabetes management in primary care* (2nd ed.). Lippincott Williams & Wilkins.
25. Lustman, P. J., & Clouse, R. E. (2005). Depression in diabetic patients: The relationship between mood and glycemic control. *Journal of Diabetes Complications., 19*, 113–122.
26. Hirschfield, R. M. A. (1999). Management of sexual side effects of antidepressant therapy. *Journal of Clinical Psychiatry, 60*(Suppl), 27–30.
27. Clayton, A. H., Pradko, J. F., Croft, H. A., et al. (2002). Prevalence of sexual dysfunction among newer antidepressants. *Journal of Clinical Psychiatry, 63*, 357–366.
28. Deshmukh, R., & Franco, K. (2003). Managing weight gain as a side effect of antidepressant therapy. *Cleveland Clinic Journal of Medicine, 70*, 614–623.
29. Morriss, R., Gask, L., Ronalds, C., et al. (1999). Clinical and patient satisfaction outcomes of a new treatment for somatized mental disorder taught to general practitioners. *British Journal of General Practice, 49*, 262–267.
30. Morriss, R. K., & Gask, L. (2002). Treatment of patients with somatized mental disorder: Effects of reattribution training on outcomes under the direct control of the family doctor. *Psychosomatics, 43*, 394–399.
31. Rosendal, M., Olesen, F., Fink, P., et al. (2007). A randomized controlled trial of brief training in the assessment and treatment of somatization in primary care: Effects on patient outcome. *General Hospital Psychiatry, 29*, 364–373.

Chapter 10
Chronic Pain

10.1 Characteristics of Pain Patients

Patients with pain cite it as the source of all their misery. They often deny the existence of other sources of emotional dysphoria and insist that their lives are blissful, except for the pain [1].

Pain not only causes emotional problems such as anxiety and depression, but also makes it difficult for patients to adapt to occupational and social lives, leading to familial conflicts, and even familial disintegration [2].

Their symptoms are likely to be prolonged when underlying psychosocial problems remain unaddressed. Therefore, the biopsychosocial aspects of pain are emphasized in its assessment and treatment.

10.2 Psychosocial Causes of Chronic Pain

Psychosocial factors, such as emotion, personality, psychodynamic, interpersonal, and behavioral factors, play an important role in pain [1].

10.2.1 Psychodynamic Factors

Patients experiencing pain without identifiable physical causes may be symbolically expressing intrapsychic conflict through their bodies. By displacing this conflict, they may feel they have a legitimate claim to have their dependency needs fulfilled [1].

Pain may also serve as a means to gain love, receive punishment for wrongdoing, or to expiate guilt [1].

K. B. Koh, *Body, Mind and Spirituality*, https://doi.org/10.1007/978-3-032-11214-9_10

It can be a response to either actual or imaginary loss and may be triggered by guilt over forbidden aggressive or sexual impulses [3].

10.2.2 Interpersonal Factors

Intractable pain has been conceptualized as a means for manipulation and gaining advantage in interpersonal relationships. For example, pain may be used to ensure the devotion of a family member or to stabilize an insecure marital relationship [1]. In this case, pain is used to reunite the patient with a person the patient wants to be close to [4].

10.2.3 Behavioral Factors

Pain behavior refers to all behaviors shown to represent that they have pain [5]. These behaviors are reinforced when rewarded, and inhibited when ignored or punished. For example, moderate pain symptoms may become intense when followed by attentive behavior of others (e.g., spouse, close family members), monetary gain, or successful avoidance of an aversive environment and distasteful activities at work [1].

Patients' complaints of severe pain despite no objective organic pathology were interpreted as their attempt to express their difficult lives. These patients often do not easily relinquish such expressions of pain [6]. Patients with self-esteem-related pain have more difficulty coping with pain psychologically than those with physical pain because patients with injury to self-esteem project their problems externally [5].

10.3 Assessment

It is important to evaluate the role of psychosocial factors in patients experiencing chronic pain [7].

10.4 Treatment

10.4.1 General Principle

Due to the multi-factorial nature of pain, various therapeutic interventions are needed [8]. First, patients with pain must be stabilized with pharmacotherapy. Then, behavioral therapy is considered to minimize pain levels. Family assessment and therapy are also required to sustain improvements in the home. Finally, for some patients, growth-oriented psychotherapy is the final step of rehabilitation. However, not all patients undergo these stages [7].

Physicians must acknowledge that the pain is real, even if psychological factors are involved. Therefore, they should use all possible therapeutic modalities, including relaxation therapy, pain education, massage, and medication [5].

It is important for physicians to maintain an optimistic attitude. While a complete cure may not be possible, various strategies can help reduce pain or distress. Physicians must guard against becoming discouraged by the patient's sense of helplessness. Treating chronic pain requires great patience [5].

Patients with chronic pain experience not only physical discomfort but also damaged self-esteem. Therefore, the techniques for interviewing these chronic pain patients are necessary for developing an effective treatment plan [5].

Patients experiencing pain should be encouraged to express their emotions. However, forcing the patients to express their emotions may prevent them from expressing their true feelings. Too much support may not only bypass the patients' psychological problems, but may actually increase conflicts related to suppression, control, and dependency [9].

Effective treatment of chronic pain improves not only pain levels but also quality of life [10].

10.4.2 Psychopharmacotherapy

Both analgesics and psychotropics are used for patients with chronic pain [11]. Antidepressants including amitriptyline and imipramine are known to be more effective than placebo in chronic pain patients [8, 12, 13]. Therapeutic effect for pain symptoms in patients with major depressive disorder requires 2-to-4 weeks of treatment with antidepressants as depression does [7, 13].

Selective serotonin receptor uptake inhibitors (SSRIs) such as fluoxetine are effective for pain relief [10]. Serotonin and noradrenalin reuptake inhibitors (SNRIs) (e.g., venlafaxine and duloxetine), which act on both serotonin and noradrenaline, appear more effective than other antidepressants in treating chronic pain [14].

In addition, antipsychotic agents such as chlorpromazine and haloperidol are sometimes used in patients with acute pain or severe pre-terminal cancer pain because these drugs potentiate the actions of narcotic analgesics [15].

10.4.3 Psychosocial Treatment

The importance of nonphysical treatments, such as psychotherapy and behavioral therapy, is emphasized due to the limitations of medication in treating chronic pain [10].

Psychotherapy

Psychotherapy begins with developing a solid psychotherapeutic alliance based on empathy. Clinicians should not confront somatizing patients with comments such as "This is all in your head." Even if pain is largely intrapsychic, it must be treated as real [1].

Patients should be told from the outset that effective pain treatment is not only performed by physicians but also requires their own efforts, and may not yield immediate results. Therefore, it should be emphasized that they should learn to live with some level of pain [16].

Clinicians should discuss the issue of psychological factors early in treatment [3]. Statements like "Pain itself may be caused by psychological problems," "Treatment should be integrative including the body and mind to be effective for pain" can be helpful [4].

Behavioral Therapy

Behavioral therapy plays an important role in the treatment of chronic pain [6]. This therapy aims to remove pain behavior and develop new behaviors incompatible with pain [17].

Behavioral therapy is subdivided into self-management and operant techniques [18].

Self-management techniques include exercise, meditation, and cognitive therapy. Operant techniques refer to treatment paradigms in which desired behavior is rewarded and undesired behavior is ignored. Mindfulness-based stress reduction (MBSR) is a mindfulness-based program that uses a combination of mindfulness meditation, body awareness, and yoga to help people become more mindful [19]. MBSR aims to help participants develop a non-judgmental awareness of moment-to-moment [20]. MBSR has been shown to reduce pain intensity and pain-related distress in patients with chronic pain (e.g., backache and joint pain) [21].

Operant approach is based on the notion that behaviors are controlled by their consequences. This model holds that behaviors persist when followed by a reward (positive reinforcement). Therefore, pain behaviors (e.g., complaints of pain and grimacing) may increase when positively reinforced [7]. In one example, when nurses withheld positive reinforcement for pain behaviors (e.g., complaints of pain), but provided attention to good behaviors (e.g., increased activity) in patients with chronic pain, they showed significant improvement.

Generally, operant approaches are used when the level of pain behavior is high despite minimal physical abnormalities. In contrast, self-management techniques are more appropriate when there is clearer evidence of tissue damage, or when operant conditioning is less effective [7].

Cognitive Behavioral Therapy

Cognitive behavioral therapy (CBT) helps patients distract themselves from pain by focusing on pleasant thoughts or sensory inputs. It may include assertiveness training and techniques to improve self-esteem and behavioral control [7].

In several studies, CBT has shown modest but sustained benefits in reducing pain, negative mood, and disability in patients with fibromyalgia, both immediately after the treatment and at long-term follow-up [22].

Traditional Psychotherapy

Traditional psychotherapy (psychodynamic therapy) is another technique that is used to treat patients with chronic pain. In particular, this psychotherapy is recommended when individuals' conflicts are prominent and behavioral changes are limited [4].

Comprehensive Approach

For patients with chronic pain, treatment should focus on the sick role. Therefore, it is desirable to place patients experiencing pain in a comprehensive pain control program or clinic where multidisciplinary modalities are available, including CBT as well as physical therapy, exercise, and vocational rehabilitation. Under such therapeutic environment, the possibility of manipulation by patients and their noncompliance can be reduced. In addition, patients with pain are more likely to accept psychological interventions in terms of integrative approach at this clinic rather than their physicians' recommendation for psychiatric treatment [1, 4].

Since it may not be possible to remove the pain, the therapeutic goal for chronic pain should be rehabilitation rather than cure [4].

Case 1

A 20-year-old male patient with end-stage renal failure was several times admitted to the department of nephrology of a general hospital to receive long-term hemodialysis. During hospitalization, he often complained of paroxysmal and severe abdominal pain. His pain was rarely relieved by either analgesics or tricyclic antidepressants. His family members could not afford to visit him, because they were busy working, but also because they were tired of taking care of him due to his chronic illness. He was therefore left alone most of the time. The nurses injected him with analgesics whenever he complained of paroxysmal abdominal pain, but he would soon complain again. He was referred to the department of psychiatry for consultation and thoroughly interviewed by a psychiatrist, who found out that the patient was afraid of coping with his illness alone, without being in his family members' care. Thereafter, the patient was interviewed for about 30 min twice every week, and his complaints of paroxysmal pain became less frequent.

This case illustrates that supportive psychotherapy can be more effective in patients with abdominal pain than medication such as analgesics and antidepressants.

Case 2

A 40-year-old male patient suffered from abdominal pain for 7 months and then underwent a variety of laboratory examinations including gastroendoscopy. However, no abnormalities were found except for signs of mild gastritis. When an internist recommended him to see a psychiatrist, the patient cast doubt on their ability to evaluate his symptoms and thereby went “doctor shopping.” No abnormal findings were found on additional physical and laboratory examinations. The patient would often lie down in his office because of severe abdominal pain, and occasionally he was absent from work. Tricyclic antidepressants were prescribed, but he continued to complain of abdominal pain, often with a grimace on his face. His pain barely improved, even after the dose of the antidepressants was increased. During an interview, the patient denied experiencing any stressors. His wife labeled him as being “egotistic” but could also not point to any significant stressors. He had been brought up by his mother as an only son, and his mother, while living with him, had never put any burden on him.

After several months, he admitted during an interview, “I get very anxious because I cannot compete with new younger employees who are good at using computers, while I am very poor at using them.” He also said, “it was a huge burden for me to attend those long-term teaching programs. I was not confident of getting good results in the post-education examinations.” After this interview, the patient gave up on getting promoted and decided to be more concerned with his own health. Since then, the intensity of his pain was markedly reduced, although he sometimes still complained of abdominal pain.

In this case, psychological factors associated with pain were revealed after having received psychiatric treatment for a considerable period of time. Therapists therefore need to be patient and wait until patients reveal such issues in the treatment of chronic pain patients, even if no psychological factors can be found at an earlier time.

10.5 Summary

1. Chronic pain may reflect hardship in life. Therefore, the assessment and treatment of chronic pain require biopsychosocial approaches.
2. Therapists need to mobilize a variety of therapeutic modalities such as psychopharmacotherapy, relaxation therapy, and cognitive behavioral therapy.
3. In particular, treatment of chronic pain requires multidisciplinary and integrative approach.
4. It is desirable for therapists to focus on rehabilitation rather than on cure as a therapeutic goal for patients with chronic pain.

5. Special therapeutic techniques are required for treatment of pain, because patients' denial of psychological problems is likely to develop resistance to psychological approach.

References

1. Sadock, B. J., & Sadock, V. A. (2003). *Synopsis of psychiatry – behavioral sciences/clinical psychiatry* (9th ed., pp. 643–660). Lippincott Williams & Wilkins.
2. Koh, K. B. (2018). *Stress and somatic symptoms: Biopsychosociospiritual perspectives* (pp. 141–156). Springer.
3. Engel, G. L. (1959). Psychogenic pain and the pain-prone patient. *American Journal of Medicine, 36*, 899–918.
4. Ford, C. V. (1984). *The somatizing disorders: Illness as a way of life* (pp. 98–126). Elsevier Biomedical.
5. Bouckoms, A., & Hackett, T. P. (1991). The pain patient: evaluation and treatment. In N. H. Cassem (Ed.), *MGH handbook of general hospital psychiatry* (3rd ed.) St. Louis: Mosby Year Book.
6. Timmermans, G., & Sternbach, R. A. (1974). Factors of human chronic pain: An analysis of personality and pain reaction variables. *Science, 184*, 806–808.
7. Houpt, J. L. (1987). Chronic pain management. In A. Soudemire & B. S. Fogel (Eds.), *Principles of medical psychiatry*. Grune & Stratton.
8. Magni, G. (1991). The use of antidepressants in the treatment of chronic pain: A review of the current evidence. *Drugs, 42*, 730–748.
9. Pilowsky, I. (1978). Pain as abnormal illness behavior. *Journal of Human Stress, 4*, 22–27.
10. Kaplan, H. I., & Sadock, B. J. (1994). *Synopsis of psychiatry: Behavioral sciences & clinical psychiatry* (7th ed., pp. 628–630, pp. 764–765) Williams & Wilkins.
11. Leigh, H., & Reiser, M. F. (1985). *The patient: Biological, psychological and social dimensions of medical practice* (2nd ed., pp. 209–240). Plenum Medical Book.
12. Onghena, P., & Van Houdenlove, B. (1992). Antidepressant induced analgesic in chronic nonmalignant pain: A meta-analysis of 39 placebo controlled studies. *Pain, 29*, 205–219.
13. Moore, D. P. (1980). Treatment of chronic pain with tricyclic antidepressants. *Southern Medical Journal, 73*, 1585–1586.
14. Somashekar, B., Jainer, A., & Wuntakal, B. (2013). Psychopharmacotherapy of somatic symptoms disorders. *International Review of Psychiatry, 25*, 107–115.
15. Goldberg, R. J., Sokol, M. S., & Cullen, L. O. (1987). Acute pain management. In: A. Soudemire & B. S. Fogel (Eds.), *Principles of medical psychiatry*. Grune & Stratton.
16. DeVaul, R. A., & Zisook, S. (1978). Chronic pain: The psychiatrist's role. *Psychosomatics, 19*, 417–421.
17. Fordyce, W. E. (1978). *Learning processes in pain*. R. A. Sternbach (Ed.), Raven Press.
18. Keefe, F. J., & Bradley, L. A. (1984). Behavioral and psychological approaches to the assessment and treatment of chronic pain. *General Hospital Psychiatry, 6*, 49–54.
19. Kabat-Zinn, J. (2013). *Full catastrophe living: Using the wisdom of your body and mind to face stress, Pain, and Illness*. Bantam Dell.
20. Schmid, S., Grossman, P., Schwarzer, B., et al. (2011). Treating fibromyalgia with mindfulness-based stress reduction: Results from a 3-armed randomized controlled trial. *Pain, 52*, 361–369.
21. Wong, S. Y., Chan, F. W., Wong, R. L., et al. (2011). Comparing the effectiveness of mindfulness-based stress reduction and multidisciplinary intervention programs for chronic pain: A randomized comparative trial. *Clinical Journal of Pain, 27*, 724–734.
22. Bernardy, K., Klose, P., & Busch, A. J., et al. (2013). Cognitive behavioral therapies for fibromyalgia. *Cochrane Database Systematic Reviews, 9*, CD009796. https://doi.org/10.1002/14651858.CD009796.pub2.

Chapter 11
Specific Somatic Symptom and Related Disorders

11.1 Somatic Symptom Disorder

11.1.1 What Is Somatic Symptom Disorder?

Somatic symptom disorder involves significant distress or functional impairment due to one or more somatic symptoms for over six months, accompanied by excessive thoughts, feelings, or behaviors related to those symptoms, regardless of whether the symptoms are medically explained. Such patients are often unresponsive to medical interventions. Some patients with this disorder are unusually sensitive to the side effects of medication [1].

11.1.2 Risk factors

The risk factors for SSD include co-occurring anxiety or depression, alexithymia [2], a history of trauma or childhood abuse/neglect [3], stressful life events [4], and personality disorders, particularly avoidant, paranoid, and obsessive-compulsive personality disorders [5].

11.1.3 Management

In patients with SSD, psychological factors associated with somatic symptoms (e.g., pain) are likely to be revealed after psychiatric treatment for a considerable period of time. Therefore, therapists need to wait patiently until patients reveal such issues and focus on rehabilitation rather than cure as the therapeutic goal for patients with SSD [6].

K. B. Koh, *Body, Mind and Spirituality*, https://doi.org/10.1007/978-3-032-11214-9_11

Various therapeutic modalities, such as psychopharmacotherapy [7], relaxation therapy [8], and cognitive behavioral therapy [9], can be used to treat patients with SSD. The management of SSD is described in detail in other chapters that address interview techniques for somatizing patients, general management of somatic symptom and related disorders, and chronic pain. A case example of SSD was presented in Chapter 10.

11.2 Illness Anxiety Disorder

11.2.1 What Is Illness Anxiety Disorder?

Illness anxiety disorder (previously called hypochondriasis) refers to a preoccupation with and fear of having a serious physical disorder over a period of six months, despite no abnormal findings and reassurance after a thorough medical evaluation [1].

Patients with illness anxiety disorder repeatedly visit their physicians with various concerns that they interpret as signs of a serious disease. They often seek medical care because they are concerned or anxious about having a specific disease rather than troubled by a specific symptom [10].

They are often emotionally constricted and have difficulty expressing themselves except through physical complaints [11, 12, 13].

11.2.2 Risk Factors

Illness anxiety disorders may sometimes be precipitated by a major life stressor or a serious but ultimately benign threat to health. Hypochondriacal symptoms may indicate somatized depression [14, 15].

11.2.3 Management

The first goal of managing patients with illness anxiety disorder is to avoid unnecessary diagnostic testing and to obviate overly aggressive medical and surgical intervention.

The second goal is to help patients cope with their symptoms, rather than trying to eliminate them completely.

Third, physicians should attempt to build durable relationships with patients based on their interest in patients as persons, not merely in their symptoms [16].

These patients are more often harmed by overaggressive than underaggressive medical management.

Therefore, the best medical interventions should be modest, simple, and benign (e.g., frequent physical examinations and vitamins). The most successful psychiatric interventions with the patients are probably cognitive, educational, and supportive [16].

Behavioral therapy and hypnosis may be useful. Psychopharmacotherapy alleviates hypochondriacal symptoms only when the patient has an underlying drug-responsive condition, such as an anxiety disorder or major depressive disorder [17].

Case

A middle-aged woman visited the department of internal medicine, being afraid of having a serious disease such as stomach cancer despite mild digestive disturbance. However, no abnormalities were found on gastroscopy. She was therefore transferred to the department of psychiatry. Her neighbor had suffered from indigestion and died several days after she was diagnosed with stomach cancer. The patient was shocked, because she experienced similar symptoms such as indigestion and abdominal discomfort. Thereafter, she began to show intolerable anxiety, guessing she might have stomach cancer, and visited a number of internists for gastric examinations, which revealed no abnormalities. Despite the physicians' reassurance, she did not accept their explanations. Rather, she was suspicious that the physicians were trying to hide the diagnosis of stomach cancer from her. She continued to be anxious for a considerable period of time after she was transferred to the department of psychiatry and treated with medications such as antianxiety and antidepressant agents as well as with supportive psychotherapy.

11.3 Functional Neurological Symptom Disorder

11.3.1 What is Functional Neurological Symptom Disorder?

Functional neurological symptom disorder (previously called conversion disorder) refers to neurological symptoms or deficits. However, the manifestations are incompatible with known pathophysiologic mechanisms or anatomic pathways [1].

The most frequent symptoms include paralysis, anesthesia, movement disorders, or sensory changes (e.g., vision and hearing) [10]. Episodes resembling epileptic seizures—also known as psychogenic or non-epileptic seizures—are also relatively common [1, 18].

Diagnosis requires that the symptoms cannot be explained by a neurological disease. This is not simply because the results of the investigations are normal or because the symptoms are bizarre. There must be clinical findings that show clear evidence of incompatibility with neurological disease [1].

Functional neurological symptom disorder may coexist with neurological disease [1]. A significant number of patients who have persistent conversion symptoms will later develop an organic disease explaining the original symptoms in retrospect [19].

While assessment of stress and trauma is important, the diagnosis should not be withheld if none is found [1].

11.3.2 Risk Factors

The potential etiological relevance of stress or trauma may be suggested by a close temporal relationship [1].

Three major theories have been proposed to explain the etiology of conversion phenomena: neurophysiologic, behavioral, and psychoanalytic theories [20].

Neurophysiological Theories

Neurophysiological theories posit inherent dysfunction in certain brain functions. For example, the disorder is basically a dysfunction of attention and recent memory due to corticofugal inhibition of afferent stimulation [21].

Behavioral Theories

Behavioral theories suggest that the patient learns to communicate feelings of helplessness and elicit environmental changes through his/her symptoms. Thus, learned helplessness during childhood can be used to manipulate and control interpersonal relationships in adulthood [22, 23]

Psychoanalytic Theories

Psychoanalytic theories stress the importance of the symbolic communication of the conversion phenomenon, and assert that the symptoms provide a compromise between the instinctual drives and their prohibitions [11, 24, 25].

11.3.3 Management

Most conversion symptoms are transient and respond to various therapeutic interventions, such as suggestive therapies (e.g., hypnosis), psychotherapy, or environmental manipulation [26]. A key therapeutic goal is to help patients discard symptoms in a face-saving manner [10].

Some persistent symptoms are perpetuated by positive reinforcers in the environment, such as family attention or financial benefits of disabilities. Patients with persistent symptoms often require intensive diagnostic and therapeutic interventions, such as inpatient psychiatric hospitalization, to extinguish this form of abnormal illness behavior [10].

When patients are resistant to psychological management, physicians can frame psychotherapy as a way to manage stress and improve coping. Hypnosis, antianxiety agents, and relaxation are effective in some cases [17].

Therapy often begins by reassuring the patient that tests revealed no physical damage, and thus recovery is expected. However, direct confrontation is rarely helpful. If symptoms persist due to chronic stress or secondary gain, resolving those issues becomes the primary goal [16].

Psychodynamic interventions, such as psychoanalysis or insight-oriented psychotherapy, help patients with functional neurological symptom disorder explore their intrapsychic conflicts and symbolism of conversion symptoms [17].

Since many stressors are interpersonal, couple or family therapy can also play a crucial role in symptom resolution [16]. The longer the duration of the patient's sick role and the more they regress, the more challenging the treatment becomes [17].

Case

A 45-year-old woman was admitted to the department of psychiatry with aphonia after no organic abnormalities were found during examinations at the ear, nose, and throat (ENT) department. At first, she was defensive, denying any stressful events. She had, however, recently learned about her husband's extramarital affair with another woman. From that moment, she was not able to pronounce anything she was trying to say. However, her symptoms rapidly improved after treatment, including supportive psychotherapy and medications such as antianxiety and antidepressant agents.

11.4 Psychological Factors Affecting Other Medical Conditions

11.4.1 What is Psychological Factors Affecting Other Medical Conditions?

The DSM-5 includes the psychological factors affecting other medical conditions (PFAOMC; previously called psychosomatic disorders) in the somatic symptom and related disorders. The essential feature of PFAOMC is the presence of one or more clinically significant psychological or behavioral factors that adversely affect the course or outcome of a medical condition. Psychological or behavioral factors include psychological distress, patterns of interpersonal interaction, coping styles, and maladaptive health behaviors, such as denial of symptoms or poor adherence to medical recommendations [1].

11.4.2 Management

Reassurance and the process of improving the patients' life situations are important during the treatment of PFAOMC. Patients with PFAOMC are usually more reluctant to deal with their emotional problems than patients with other psychiatric problems. Therefore, psychiatrists must focus the therapy on understanding the motivations and mechanisms of disturbed functioning and helping patients realize the nature of their illness and the implications of its costly adaptive patterns. These insights can lead to changed and healthier behavioral patterns [17].

Family therapy is helpful for patients with PFAOMC. This therapy offers the hope of a change in the relationship between family members who are often mentally stressed and reactively hostile toward the sick members. In addition, relaxation techniques, hypnosis, and biofeedback can be used for these patients [17].

The management of PFAOMC is described in other chapters that address individual physical diseases and functional physical disorders.

11.5 Factitious Disorder

11.5.1 What is Factitious Disorder?

Factitious disorder is an illness in which patients artificially produce symptoms themselves in the absence of obvious external rewards and seek sick roles. In most cases, individuals with factitious disorder present with somatic symptoms [1].

The underlying motivation of factitious disorder is believed to stem from intrapsychic or interpersonal reasons [10].

Malingering is differentiated from factitious disorder by the intentional reporting of symptoms for external gains (e.g., to obtain disability or compensation payments or to avoid conscription into military service) [1].

11.5.2 Management

No specific psychiatric therapy is effective for patients with factitious disorder. Thus, treatment is best focused on management rather than on cure.

Clinicians must recognize that even though the patient's illness is factitious, the patient is ill [17].

The therapeutic approach to factitious disorder begins with confronting the patient with the physician's knowledge of the behavior. This can be done in a supportive manner that conveys the physician's concern for the patient and willingness to be helpful [27].

Occasionally, some patients with factitious disorder have an underlying depression. These patients' prognosis is better because depression is a treatable disorder [10].

Psychopharmacotherapy of factitious disorder is of limited use. Selective serotonin reuptake inhibitors (SSRIs) may be useful in decreasing impulsive behaviors in acting-out factitious behavior [17].

Case

A 65-year-old woman was admitted to the eye department of a general hospital with sudden loss of vision, but physical and neurological examinations did not reveal any abnormalities. She was therefore transferred to the department of psychiatry. She did not complain of anything except her loss of vision. However, she seemed indifferent and defensive, not expressing her feelings for a considerable period of time. Later, one of her family members revealed that she had experienced a serious conflict with her son-in-law due to economic problems. When he asked her to lend him money, she refused. Thereafter, he avoided her eyes whenever he met her while they were living in the same house. Supportive psychotherapy and medication, including the antianxiety agent ethyl loflazepate and the antidepressant amitriptyline, did not improve her symptoms. After being discharged from the hospital without improvement, the patient continued to complain of her loss of vision when visiting the outpatient department; she was not able to see the knob in front of the door when leaving the room after the interview was finished. However, at home she was found picking up hair in her room by a family member.

This case was initially considered functional neurological symptom disorder, but later diagnosed as factitious disorder, because she was found to artificially produce symptoms herself in the absence of external rewards.

11.6 Summary

1. This section reviewed the assessment, risk factors, and management associated with somatic symptom-related disorders, such as somatic symptom disorder, illness anxiety disorder, functional neurological symptom disorder, psychological factors affecting other medical conditions (PFAOMC), and factitious disorder.
2. Case examples were presented for illness anxiety disorder (hypochondriasis), functional neurological symptom disorder (conversion disorder), and factitious disorder.

References

1. American Psychiatric Association (APA). (2013). *Statistical and diagnostic manual of mental disorders* (5th ed.). Am Psychiatric Publishing.
2. Smakowski, A., Hüsing, P., & Völcker, S. et al. (2024). Psychological risk factors of somatic symptom disorder: A systematic review and meta-analysis of cross-sectional and longitudinal studies. *Journal of Psychosomatic Research, 181*, 111608. https://doi.org/10.1016/j.jpsychores.2024.111608.
3. Kurlansik, S. L., & Maffei, M. S. (2016). Somatic symptom disorder. *American Family Physician, 93*, 49–54.
4. Harris, A. M., Orav, E. J., Bates, D. W., et al. (2009). Somatization increases disability independent of comorbidity. *Journal of General Internal Medicine, 24*, 155–161.
5. Rost, K. M., Akins, R. N., Brown, F. W., et al. (1992). The comorbidity of DSM-III-R personality disorders in somatization disorder. *General Hospital Psychiatry, 14*, 322–326.
6. Ford, C. V. (1984). *The somatizing disorders: Illness as a way of life* (pp. 98–126). Elsevier Biomedical.
7. Somashekar, B., Jainer, A., & Wuntakal, B. (2013). Psychopharmacotherapy of somatic symptoms disorders. *International Review of Psychiatry, 25*, 107–115.
8. Bouckoms, A., & Hackett, T. P. (1991). The pain patient: evaluation and treatment. In N. H. Cassem (Ed.), *MGH handbook of general hospital psychiatry* (3rd ed.). Mosby Year Book.
9. Bernardy, K., Klose, P., & Busch, A. J. et al. (2013). Cognitive behavioral therapies for fibromyalgia. *Cochrane Database Systematic Reviews, 9*, CD009796. https://doi.org/10.1002/14651858.CD009796.pub2
10. Ford, C. V., & Smith, G. R. Jr. (1987). Somatoform disorders, factitious disorder, and disability syndromes. In A. Stoudemire & B. S. Fogel (Eds.), *Principles of medical psychiatry*. Grune & Stratton.
11. Ford, C. V. (1983). *The somatizing disorders: Illness as a way of life*. Elsevier.
12. Kenyon, F. E. (1965). Hypochondriasis: A survey of some historical, clinical and social aspects. *British Journal of Medical Psychology, 38*, 117–133.
13. Pilowsky, I. (1970). Primary and secondary hypochondriasis. *Acta Psychiatrica Scandinavica, 47*, 484–509.
14. Katon, W., Kleinman, A., & Rosen, G. (1982). Depression and somatization: A review (part 1). *American Journal of Medicine, 72*, 127–135.
15. Katon, W., Kleinman, A., & Rosen, G. (1982). Depression and somatization: A review (part 2). *American Journal of Medicine, 72*, 241–247.
16. Cassem, N. H., & Barsky, A. J. (1991) Functional somatic symptoms and somatoform disorders. In N. H. Cassem (Ed.), *MGH handbook of general hospital psychiatry* (3ed ed.). Mosby Year Book.
17. Sadock, B. J., & Sadock, V. A. (2003). *Synopsis of psychiatry – behavioral sciences/clinical psychiatry* (9th ed.). Lippincott Williams & Wilkins.
18. Tilahun, B. B. S., & Bautista, J. F. (2022). Psychogenic nonepileptic seizure: An empathetic, practical approach. *Cleveland Clinic Journal of Medicine, 89*, 252–259.
19. Watson, C. G., & Buranen, C. (1979). The frequency and identification of false positive conversion reactions. *Journal of Nervous and Mental Disease, 167*, 243–247.
20. Jones, M. M. (1980). Conversion reaction: Anacronism or evolutionary form: A review of the neurologic, behavioral, and psychoanalytic literature. *Psychological Bulletin, 87*, 427–441.
21. Ludwig, A. M. (1972). Hysteria: A neurobiological theory. *Archives of General Psychiatry, 27*, 771–777.
22. Halleck, S. L. (1967). Hysterical personality traits. *Archives of General Psychiatry, 16*, 750–757.
23. Celani, D. (1976). An interpersonal approach to hysteria. *American Journal of Psychiatry, 133*, 1414–1418.
24. Hollender, M. H. (1972). Conversion hysteria: A post-Freudian reinterpretation of 19th century psychosocial data. *Archives of General Psychiatry, 26*, 311–314.

25. Hollender, M. H. (1976). Hysteria. The culture-bound syndromes. *Papua New Guinea Medical Journal, 19*, 24–29.
26. Folks, D. G., Ford, C. V., & Regan, W. M. (1984). Conversion symptoms in a general hospital. *Psychosomatics, 25*, 285–295.
27. Hollander, M. H., & Hersh, S. P. (1970). Impossible consultation made possible. *Archives of General Psychiatry, 23*, 343–345.

Part IV
Resilience-Enhancing Approaches to Physical Diseases

Chapter 12
Depression in the Medically Ill

12.1 Screening for Depression in Medically Ill Patients

Despite the difficulties in screening for depression in medically ill patients due to the overlap of symptoms between medical and depressive conditions, it is important to recognize and treat depression in this population. Doing so can significantly improve quality of life [1] and positively influence the outcomes of physical illnesses [2].

12.2 Outcomes of Comorbid Depression in the Medically Ill

Depression can exacerbate physical illnesses, contributing to mortality rates higher than those expected from the physical illness alone [3, 4].

12.3 Relationship between Physical Diseases and Depression

Depression can manifest itself as symptoms related to either physical diseases or medication, responses to physical diseases, and comorbidity of physical diseases and psychiatric disorders [5, 6, 7].

K. B. Koh, *Body, Mind and Spirituality*, https://doi.org/10.1007/978-3-032-11214-9_12

12.4 Emotional Reaction to the Diagnosis of a Chronic Illness

The emotional reaction to the diagnosis of a chronic illness can be a greater challenge than coping with the physical manifestations of the illness [8].

12.5 Psychodynamics of Depression in the Medically Ill

Medically ill patients are likely to be depressed because their physical diseases can increase existing conflicts and vulnerabilities. In particular, a sense of loss is a common experience observed in patients with serious medical conditions [9, 10], and decreased self-esteem plays a central role in the development of depression [11].

12.6 Why Do Physicians Miss Depression in the Medically Ill?

Physicians may misattribute depressive symptoms to the physical illness itself. For example, somatic symptoms such as poor appetite, weight loss, fatigue, and insomnia are noted in both physical and depressive disorders.

Additionally, depression is often seen as a normal response to physical illness. For accurate differential diagnoses, physicians must focus more on psychological symptoms—such as anhedonia (loss of pleasure or interest), hopelessness, crying, guilt, reduced self-esteem, unworthiness, and suicidal ideation—than on physical symptoms [12].

12.7 Clinical Evaluation of Depression

Clinicians should pay particular attention to the psychological symptoms of depression like anhedonia (loss of pleasure or interest) in medically ill patients. Personal and family histories of the patients are also important, as a previous history of major depressive disorder can increase the likelihood of a current depressive episode [13, 14].

12.8 Evaluation of Major Psychological Symptoms in Depressed Patients with Physical Diseases

12.8.1 Depressed Mood and Anhedonia

Assessing interest or pleasure in medically ill patients can be challenging. Older patients show a sense of hopelessness and helplessness instead of depressed mood or anhedonia. These feelings are regarded as being identical to depression. Avoidance of others and disinterest in self-care or other activities can indicate anhedonia [15].

12.8.2 Feelings of Unworthiness and Excessive Guilt

Patients with major depressive disorder have bad feelings about themselves rather than situations. For example, they may express their unworthiness by saying, "I am bad, " whereas they express their self-reproach by saying, "I am bad because I am a burden." They express excessive or inappropriate guilt by saying, "It is a punishment that I am ill" [15, 16].

12.8.3 Suicidal Ideation

While patients with major depressive disorder often experience persistent suicidal thoughts, patients with severe physical illness may express a desire to die due to overwhelming pain. In these cases, such expressions may be interpreted as logical or even understandable by caregivers and physicians. However, such statements should not be immediately equated with suicidal ideation and must be assessed in context [17].

12.9 Biopsychosocial Evaluation

Biopsychosocial evaluation should precede treatment of depression in the medically ill [6].

12.9.1 Use of Psychological Instruments

The Beck Depression Inventory is useful for screening depression, whereas the Hamilton Rating Scale for Depression is useful for screening and evaluating the degree of depression [18].

12.9.2 Find out Precipitating Factors of Depression

The presence and absence of social support, adaptation to job, family roles, sexual functioning, body image, and the personal meaning of illness should be checked [6].

12.9.3 Identify Physical Diseases and Medications Related to Depression

Mood disorders associated with medical conditions or medications are similar to major depressive disorder in presentation but have organic causes [19]. Physical diseases and medications commonly associated with depression include the following [1, 20]:

Physical Diseases

Cancer (brain and pancreatic cancer), stroke, systemic lupus erythematosus (SLE), chronic obstructive pulmonary disease (COPD), endocrine diseases (hypothyroidism, Cushing's syndrome, hypoglycemia), lymphoma, Parkinson's disease, pernicious anemia (vitamin B12 deficiency), viral infections (influenza, hepatitis, mononucleosis, Epstein-Barr virus), coronary heart disease, and end-stage renal disease, among others.

Medications

Antihypertensives (reserpine, propranolol, methyldopa), barbiturates, cimetidine, corticosteroids, levodopa, benzodiazepines, diuretics (e.g., thiazides, spironolactone), and clonidine, among others.

According to the DSM-5, depression associated with medications is termed "substance/medication-induced depressive disorder", whereas mood symptoms arising from medical conditions fall under "depressive disorder due to another medical condition" [20].

The treatment of mood disorders due to medical conditions should begin with the treatment of the underlying physical disease or discontinuing the offending medication. However, in cases where the physical disease cannot be treated or medication cannot be discontinued, clinicians should cautiously initiate the biopsychosocial approach used in the treatment of major depressive disorder without organic causes [20].

12.10 Psychosocial Treatment

Psychosocial treatment for depressed patients with physical diseases differs from the treatment used for patients with primary depression.

12.10.1 Resistance to Psychiatric Intervention in Depressive Patients with Physical Diseases

Patients with physical diseases and depression often deny depression and refuse to visit psychiatrists. They may feel angry and humiliated when primary physicians perceive their problems as psychiatric rather than physical. In such cases, physicians find it difficult to perform diagnostic evaluations or provide psychotherapy. Initial conversations should begin with empathy regarding the patients' anger and frustration [21], similar to approaches used for somatizing patients [22].

12.10.2 Depression Consequent to Serious Illness

Depression has been conceptualized as a response to narcissistic injury [23]. In any serious illness, the mind sustains an injury of its own, as though an illness, for example myocardial infarction (MI), produces ego infarction [24].

Management of Acute Depression

Illness-induced depression can disrupt work and interpersonal relationships [25]. Physicians should focus on preserving patients' sense of self-esteem. Even patients with strong recovery potential may be vulnerable to self-esteem injury. It is important to help patients feel unique and appreciated by asking personal questions [24].

Management of Chronic Depression

Patients who return home from hospital often report feeling weak and emotionally low. This phenomenon is sometimes termed "homecoming depression" [26]. However, a large portion of this weakness is due to muscular atrophy and the systemic effects of immobilization [24].

Occasionally, patients may feel afraid of leaving their homes, perceiving routine activities such as walking as too dangerous [24]. The best treatment for psychological constriction is a program that emphasizes early and progressive mobilization in hospitals, followed by continued exercise after discharge [27, 28, 29, 30]. Even when physical recovery is limited, it should be emphasized that psychological rehabilitation is still possible [24].

Therapeutic staff, including physicians, should adopt a supportive stance, presenting themselves as consultants rather than authoritarian figures [31]. Empathetic listening, especially with uncooperative patients, allows for emotional ventilation and facilitates better regulation of their emotional reactions to illnesses, such as anxiety, depression, anger, and guilt.

In diabetes education, especially regarding diet, it is desirable to help patients change maladaptive habits through supportive strategies rather than use coercion [32]. Diabetes can be exacerbated by stressors; therefore, it is important to identify stressors and seek psychiatric consultation, if necessary. Psychiatric consultation is recommended when severe depression is noted [32]. Moreover, for depressed patients with feelings of hopelessness and helplessness, physicians need to minimize the injury to patients' self-esteem rather than manage diabetes itself (e.g., dietary compliance) [33], as shown in the following case.

Case

A 40-year-old woman with diabetes hospitalized in the department of endocrinology was referred to the department of psychiatry for management of uncontrolled eating. She had suffered from diabetes for a period of 10 years and had difficulty walking due to complications such as peripheral neuropathy. After realizing that diabetes could not be cured completely while reading a pamphlet on the illness, she began to live in a state of self-abandonment, feeling a sense of hopelessness and helplessness. Thereafter, she gave up her diet and ate sweet foods such as cakes and doughnuts carelessly. The internist reproached her for not complying with his diet requests when her blood sugar levels rose above 400 mg/dl even after insulin had been injected several times during her admission. She cried out, saying, "any patient who can control their eating is not a real diabetic patient." After venting her emotions such as anger and resentment toward the physician, the psychiatrist said, "please eat as many doughnuts as you can now, but start trying to cut down on the number one by one." The patient calmed down after that. Later, she followed the internist's diet advice and did not buy any more sweet foods at the cafeteria of the hospital. She also looked peaceful and emotionally stable, reading the Bible in her room.

12.11 Biological Treatment: Antidepressants in the Medically Ill

12.11.1 General Principle

A biological model in which psychopharmacological agents correct chemical imbalances related to depression in medically ill patients can help clinicians establish therapeutic relationships with patients who are resistant to psychological approaches. Ultimately, patients should be approached using a biopsychosocial model [21].

12.11.2 Drug–Disease and Drug–Drug Interactions

Prior to administering antidepressants to medically ill patients, clinicians should answer the following three questions [12]:

First, does the physical disease affect drug metabolism?

Patients with liver disease cannot effectively metabolize antidepressants. Renal disease reduces the clearance of antidepressants. Therefore, clinicians should start using low doses of antidepressants in patients with renal and liver diseases.

Second, does the drug affect the physical disease?

Tricyclic antidepressants can increase post-myocardial infarction mortality [34]. These drugs cause severe orthostatic hypotension in patients with congestive heart failure. Trazodone can cause arrhythmia in patients with unstable cardiac conditions [35]. Antidepressants that block dopamine receptors can exacerbate Parkinson's disease, whereas dopamine agonists can improve the disease. Because Alzheimer disease is linked to choline system abnormalities, drugs with anticholinergic effects can exacerbate the disease [12].

Third, is there the possibility of drug–drug interactions?

Tricyclic antidepressants can block the antihypertensive effects of clonidine, methyldopa, and guanethidine while enhancing the effect of prazosin [36].

Among the selective serotonin reuptake inhibitors (SSRIs), sertraline is the most preferred drug in terms of drug–drug interactions due to its minimal inhibition of cytochrome P450 IID6 [37].

12.12 Use of Antidepressants in Specific Physical Diseases

This section reviews the use of antidepressants in patients with cardiac, renal, hepatic, and respiratory diseases, as well as diabetes, and insomnia. The use of antidepressants in patients with other disorders, such as chronic pain, gastrointestinal diseases, stroke, and cancer, has been discussed in other chapters. The dosages and main side effects of the antidepressants used in adults and older patients are described in Table 12.1 [38].

12.12.1 Cardiac Diseases

Antidepressants, such as selective serotonin reuptake inhibitors (SSRIs), bupropion, and venlafaxine, can be used instead of tricyclics because they do not produce cardiovascular side effects, including orthostatic hypotension [39, 40].

Sertraline is considered a safe drug because it does not significantly interact with digoxin [41].

In general, sertraline and citalopram are recommended as first-line pharmacotherapy for depression, especially major depressive disorder, in patients with coronary heart disease (CHD) or congestive heart failure. Mirtazapine, bupropion, venlafaxine, and tricyclic antidepressants should be viewed as second- or third-line treatment options [42].

12.12.2 Renal Diseases

SSRIs such as fluoxetine are not significantly affected by renal function disturbances [43, 44]. However, the half-life of venlafaxine in patients with renal disease is considerably longer and its clearance rate is somewhat lower. Therefore, this drug should be started at a low dose and gradually increased [45].

12.12.3 Hepatic Diseases

Patients with liver disease often exhibit hypersensitivity to the sedative effects of psychotropics [46]. Therefore, it is desirable to use antidepressants with low sedative action to treat insomnia in patients with liver disease [47]. Sertraline, which has a shorter half-life, is better than fluoxetine for the treatment of depression associated with liver disease [48].

12.12.4 Respiratory Diseases

Tricyclic antidepressants such as imipramine and SSRIs such as citalopram are known to improve the status of asthma as well as depression in patients with comorbid

Table 12.1 The dosages and side effects of antidepressants

	Daily doses of adults (older patients)(mg)	Main side effects
TCAs		
Amitriptyline(Elavil)	20 ~ 200(10 ~ 75)	Drowsiness, dry mouth, constipation, difficulty in urination, edema, blurred vision, increased appetite, weight gain, orthostatic hypotension, mania, seizure
Imipramine(Tofranil)	50 ~ 200(25 ~ 75)	Same as above
Nortriptyline(Aventyl)	30 ~ 150(30 ~ 50)	Increased blood pressure, numbness, dry mouth, nausea, vomiting, decreased appetite, blurred vision, rash
SARIs		
Trazodone(Trittico)	50 ~ 250 (25 ~ 75)	Drowsiness, orthostatic hypotension, dizziness, headache, nausea, priapism
Nefazodone(Serzone)	100 ~ 300 (50 ~ 200)	Orthostatic hypotension
SSRIs		
Fluoxetine(Prozac)	20–60(10 ~ 20)	Nausea, vomiting, diarrhea, abdominal pain, decreased appetite (early), headache, insomnia, anxiety, tremor, hidrosis, decreased sexual desire
Sertraline(Zoloft)	50–200(25 ~ 75)	Same as above
Fluvoxamine(Luvox)	50–200(25 ~ 75)	Same as above
Paroxetine(Paxil)	20 ~ 60(10 ~ 20)	Myoclonus, dry mouth in addition to the above
Escitalopram(Lexapro)	10 ~ 20(5 ~ 15)	Same as above
SNRIs		
Venlafaxine(Effexor)	75 ~ 225(25 ~ 75)	Drowsiness, dizziness, nausea, dry mouth, constipation, decreased appetite, listlessness, anxiety, impotence
Duloxetine(Cymbalta)	60 ~ 120(30 ~ 60)	Nausea, dry mouth, insomnia, increased blood pressure
Milnacipran(Ixel)	25 ~ 100(10 ~ 50)	Nausea, vomiting, constipation, stomach pain, weight loss, dry mouth, headache
NaSSAs		
Mirtazapine(Remeron)	15 ~ 45(7.5 ~ 15)	Drowsiness, dizziness, dry mouth, constipation, Edema, increased appetite, weight gain
NDRIs		
Bupropion(Wellbutrin)	150 ~ 300(75 ~ 100)	Headache, insomnia, nausea, restlessness, seizure

(continued)

Table 12.1 (continued)

	Daily doses of adults (older patients)(mg)	Main side effects
SSREs		
Tianeptine(Stablon)	25 ~ 37.5(25)	Drowsiness, headache, dizziness, dry mouth, nausea, constipation, decreased appetite, tachycardia, listlessness, tremor

TCAs: Tricyclic antidepressants, SARIs: Serotonin antagonist and reuptake inhibitors, SSRIs: Selective serotonin reuptake inhibitors, SNRIs: Serotonin-norepinephrine reuptake inhibitors, NaSSAs: Noradrenergic and specific serotonergic antidepressants, NDRIs: norepinephrine-dopamine reuptake inhibitors, SSREs: Selective serotonin reuptake enhancers.

bronchial asthma and depression [49, 50]. As with benzodiazepines, the antidepressant dose may need to be lower in these patients than in those without physical diseases [49].

Less sedating antidepressants should be used in patients with compromised pulmonary status (e.g., COPD and sleep apnea) to prevent respiratory depression [51, 52].

12.12.5 Diabetes

SSRIs and serotonin norepinephrine reuptake inhibitors (SNRIs), such as duloxetine and venlafaxine, are the most appropriate antidepressants for managing depression in patients with diabetes because of their favorable side effects [53]. However, certain antidepressants should be used with caution. For example, SSRIs, such as fluoxetine, sertraline, and paroxetine, may cause hypoglycemia [54]. Tricyclic antidepressants, such as imipramine, may cause hypoglycemia when used for a brief period but hyperglycemia when used for a long-term period [55].

To prevent side effects (e.g., anxiety and restlessness) and the recurrence of depression, antidepressant medications should not be discontinued abruptly under any circumstances. Medications should be tapered slowly over a 1- to 2-week period [56, 57].

Among antidepressants, SSRIs and venlafaxine are more likely to cause sexual dysfunction than bupropion or duloxetine [58].

Moreover, weight gain may occur with the use of antidepressants in patients with diabetes [56]. In particular, tricyclic antidepressants such as amitriptyline and SSRIs such as paroxetine can cause weight gain. Fluoxetine may cause weight loss when used for less than 6 months but weight gain when used for more than 6 months [59]. To manage weight gain associated with antidepressant treatment, patients are recommended to improve their diet and initiate exercise programs, and the medication should be changed to weight-neutral medications (e.g., duloxetine and bupropion).

12.12.6 *Sleep Disorders*

For sleep disorders in patients with depression and physical illness, the use of antidepressants with sedative action, rather than the combined use of antidepressants and hypnotics, may prevent complications caused by medications. Sedative action is more potent in tricyclic antidepressants (e.g., amitriptyline), mirtazapine, and trazodone than in SSRIs (e.g., sertraline), venlafaxine, and bupropion [40, 60, 61, 62].

12.12.7 *Other Symptoms*

Tricyclic antidepressants are used to treat conditions other than depression. These conditions include enuresis, chronic pain, migraine, and peptic ulcer. Tricyclic antidepressants can have a dual effect in patients with depression and the aforementioned physical symptoms. SSRIs have also been used effectively to treat chronic pain and migraine [12].

Tricyclic antidepressants should be avoided in patients with a history of eye disease, because their anticholinergic effects can facilitate narrow-angle glaucoma. However,SSRIs can be safely administered to patients with glaucoma. SSRIs, bupropion, and venlafaxine are recommended over tricyclic antidepressants or MAO inhibitors in patients with depression andobesity because they do not cause weight gain [12].

12.13 Therapeutic Interventions

Cognitive behavioral therapy, physical rehabilitation, and antidepressant treatment have positive impacts on the quality of life as well as mood in depressed patients with physical diseases (e.g., COPD) [1, 63, 64, 65].

Complex psychological and/or lifestyle interventions that includeexercise significantly improve the symptoms of depression in patients with COPD [66]. In addition, various treatment modalities, including medication, psychotherapy, social support, and spiritual intervention, need to be considered for the management of depression in medically ill patients. Therefore, clinicians' therapeutic approaches should be tailored to the specific needs of such patients from a biopsychosocial perspective [67].

12.14 Summary

1. For treatment of depression in the medically ill, addressing underlying organic causes is paramount.
2. Therapists should address patients' resistance to psychiatric approach and depressive reaction to severe physical illness.
3. It is important to choose appropriate antidepressants as a biological treatment. Therapists also need to pay attention to drug–disease and drug–drug interactions.
4. Antidepressants, such as selective serotonin reuptake inhibitors (SSRIs), bupropion, and venlafaxine, are effective in treating depression in medically ill patients. However, tricyclic antidepressants can still be effectively used for patients experiencing pain.
5. The psychosocial approach for medically ill patients with depression should be supportive, allowing them to ventilate their emotions, minimizing injury to self-esteem, and fostering hope.
6. Therapeutic staff, including physicians, should engage patients with warmth and partnership as consultants, avoiding authoritarian attitudes.
7. Even when physical recovery is limited, it should be emphasized that psychological recovery remains possible.
8. Clinicians' therapeutic approaches should be tailored to the specific needs of patients from a biopsychosociospiritual perspective.

References

1. Wilson, I. (2006). Depression in the patient with COPD. *International Journal of Chronic Obstructive Pulmonary Disease, 1*, 61–64.
2. Ng, T. P., Niti, M., Tan, W. C., et al. (2007). Depressive symptoms and chronic obstructive pulmonary disease: Effect on mortality, hospital readmission, symptom burden, functional status, and quality of life. *Archives of Internal Medicine, 167*, 60–67.
3. Katon, W., & Sullivan, M. D. (1990). Depression and chronic medical illness. *The Journal of Clinical Psychiatry, 51*(Suppl 6), 3–11.
4. Rovner, B. W., German, P. S., & Brant, L. J. (1991). Depression and mortality in nursing homes. *JAMA, 265*, 993–996.
5. Hall, R. C. W. (1980). *Depression in psychiatric presentations of medical illness: Somatopsychic disorders*. SP Medical & Scientific Books.
6. Rodin, G., & Voshart, K. (1986). Depression in the medically ill: An overview. *The American Journal of Psychiatry, 143*, 696–705.
7. Duric, V., Clayton, S., Leong, M. L., et al. (2016). Comorbidity factors and brain mechanisms linking chronic stress and systemic illness. *Neural Plasticity*, 5460732. https://doi.org/10.1155/2016/5460732. Epub 2016 Feb 8.
8. Lewis, K. S. (1998). Emotional adjustment to a chronic illness. *Lippincott's Primary Care Practice, 2*, 38–51.
9. Freud S. Mourning and melancholia. In: Jones E, editor. Collected papers. Vol 4. 1950.London: Hogarth Press; 1917.
10. Spitz, R. (1942). Anaclitic depression: An inquiry into the genesis of psychiatric conditions in early childhood. *The Psychoanalytic Study of the Child, 2*, 313–342.

11. Bibring, E. (1965). The mechanism of depression. In P. Greenacre (Ed.), *Affective disorders*. International Universities Press.
12. Cohen-Cole, S. A., Brown, F. W., & McDaniel, J. S. (1993). Assessment of depression and grief reactions in the medically ill. In A. Stoudemire & B. S. Fogel (Eds.), *Psychiatric care of the medical patient*. Oxford University Press.
13. Akiskal, H. S., Djenderedjian, A. H., & Bolinger, J. M. (1978). The joint use of clinical and biological criteria for psychiatric diagnosis. In H. S. Akiskal & W. L. Webb (Eds.), *Psychiatric diagnosis: Exploration of biological predictors*. Spectrum Publications.
14. Hirschfeld, R. M. A., Koslow, S. H., & Kupfer, D. J. (1983). The clinical utility of the dexamethasone suppression test in psychiatry. *J Am Med Ass, 250*, 2172.
15. Cavanaugh, S. (1991). Depression in the medically ill. In F. K. Judd, G. D. Burrows, & D. R. Lipsitt (Eds.), *Handbook of studies on general hospital psychiatry*. Elsevier Science Publishers BV (Biomedical Division).
16. Cavanaugh, S., Clark, D., & Gibbons, R. (1983). Diagnosing depression in the hospitalized medically ill. *Psychosomatics, 24*, 809–815.
17. Cavanaugh, S. (1995). Depression in the medically ill: Critical issues in diagnostic assessment. *Psychosomatics, 36*, 48–59.
18. Yang, C. K., Woo, C. H., & Han, H. M. (1992). A study on depression in medical inpatients. *Journal of Korean Neuropsychiatric Association, 31*, 1073–1083.
19. Stoudemire A. Selected organic brain syndromes. In: Hales R, Yudofski, editors. Textbook of neuropsychiatry.: APA Press; 1987.
20. Cohen-Cole, S. A., & Harpe, C. (1987). Diagnostic assessment of depression in the medically ill. In A. Stoudemire & B. S. Fogel (Eds.), *Principles of medical psychiatry*. Orlando.
21. Keller, M., Klerman, G., & Lavori, P. (1982). Treatment received by depressed patients. *JAMA, 248*, 1848–1855.
22. Koh, K. B. (2013). An effective approach to somatization assessment and management. In K. B. Koh (Ed.), *Somatization and psychosomatic symptoms* (pp. 99–111). Springer.
23. Bibring, E. (1953). The mechanism of depression. In P. Greenacre (Ed.), *Affective disorders: Psychoanalytic contributions to their study*. International Universities Press.
24. Cassem, N. H. (1991). Depression. In N. H. Cassem (Ed.), *MGH handbook of general hospital psychiatry* (3d ed.). Mosby Year Book.
25. Cassem, N. H., & Hackett, T. P. (1971). Psychiatric consultation in a coronary care unit. *Annals of Internal Medicine, 75*, 9–14.
26. Wishnie, H. A., Hackett, T. P., & Cassem, N. H. (1971). Psychologic hazards of convalescence following myocardial infarction. *JAMA, 215*, 1292–1296.
27. Andrews, J. L., Jr. (1986). *Pulmonary rehabilitation. Pract Cardiol, 12*, 127–137.
28. Gift, A. G., Plaut, S. M., & Jacox, A. (1986). Psychologic and physiologic factors related to dyspnea in subjects with chronic obstructive pulmonary disease. *Heart & Lung, 15*, 595–602.
29. Pardy, R. L., Rivington, R. N., & Despas, P. J. (1981). Inspiratory muscle training compared with physiotherapy in patients with chronic airflow limitation. *The American Review of Respiratory Disease, 123*, 421–425.
30. Unger, K. M., Moser, K. M., & Hanser, P. (1980). Selection of an exercise program for patients with chronic obstructive pulmonary disease. *Heart & Lung, 9*, 68–76.
31. Kimball, C. P. (1981). *The biopsychosocial approach to the patient*. Williams & Wilkins.
32. Koh, K. B. (2011). *Stress and psychosomatic medicine* (2nd ed.). Ilchokak.
33. Koh, K. B., & Bae, J. H. (1988). Coping strategy of patients with diabetes mellitus. *Journal of Korean Neuropsychiatric Association, 27*, 685–692.
34. Glassman, A. H., Roose, S. P., & Bigger, J. T. (1993). The safety of tricyclic antidepressants in cardiac patients [letter]. *JAMA, 269*, 2673–2675.
35. Janowsky, D., Curtis, G., & Zisook, S. (1983). Ventricular arrhythmias possibly aggravated by trazodone. *The American Journal of Psychiatry, 140*, 796–797.
36. Crewe HK, Lennard MS. Tucker GT. The effect of paroxetine and other specific serotonin reuptake inhibitors on cytochrome P450IID6 activity in human liver microsomes. British Journal of Clinical Pharmacology 1991;32:658–659.

37. Preskorn, S. H. (1993). Phamacokinetics of antidepressants: Why and how they are relevant to treatment. *The Journal of Clinical Psychiatry, 54*(Suppl 9), 14–34.
38. Koh, K. B. (2018). *Stress and somatic symptoms: Biopsychosociospiritual perspectives*. Springer.
39. Katon, W., Sullivan, M., & Clark, M. (1995). Cardiovascular Disorders. In H. I. Kaplan & B. J. Sadock (Eds.), *Comprehensive textbook of psychiatry* (6th ed.). Williams & Wilkins.
40. McElroy, S. L., Keck, P. E., & Friedman, L. M. (1995). Minimizing and managing antidepressant side-effects. *The Journal of Clinical Psychiatry, 56*(Suppl 2), 49–55.
41. Warrington, S. J. (1991). Clinical implications of the pharmacology of sertraline. *International Clinical Psychopharmacology, 6*(Suppl 2), 11–21.
42. Shapiro, P. (2009). Psychopharmacology in cardiac disease. In S. Ferrando, J. Levenson, M. Robinson, et al. (Eds.), *Handbook of psychopharmacology in the medically ill*. American Psychiatric Publishing.
43. Aronoff, G. R., Bergstrom, R. F., & Pottratz, S. T. (1984). Fluoxetine kinetics and protein binding in normal and impaired renal function. *Clinical Pharmacology and Therapeutics, 36*, 138–144.
44. Bergstrom, R. F., Beasley, C. M., & Levy, N. B. (1993). The effects of renal and hepatic disease on the pharmacokinetics, renal tolerance, and risk-benefit profile of fluoxetine. *International Clinical Psychopharmacology, 8*, 261–266.
45. Stoudemire, A., & Fogel, B. S. (1995). Psychopharmacology in medical patients: An update. In A. Stoudemire & B. S. Fogel (Eds.), *Medical-psychiatric practice* (Vol. 3). American Psychiatric Press.
46. Holm, E., Uhl, W., & Stamm, S. (1986). Safety of fluvoxamine for patients with chronic liver disease: Biochemical variables, psychometric performance and EEG. *Advances in Pharmacotherapy, 2*, 151–165.
47. Beliles, K., & Stoudemire, A. (1998). Psychopharmacologic treatment of depression in the medically ill. *Psychosomatics, 39*, S2–S19.
48. Beliles, K. E., & Stoudemire, A. (1995). Psychopharmacokinetics: Clinical applications in medical illnesses. In A. Stoudemire & B. S. Fogel (Eds.), *Medical psychiatric practice* (Vol. 3). American Psychiatric Press Inc.
49. Thompson, W. L., & Thompson, T. L., II. (1987). Pulmonary disease. In A. Stoudemire & B. S. Fogel (Eds.), *Principles of medical psychiatry*. Grune & Stratton.
50. Brown, E. S., Vigil, L., Khan, D. A., Liggin, J. D., et al. (2005). A randomized trial of citalopram versus placebo in outpatients with asthma and major depressive disorder: A proof of concept study. *Biological Psychiatry, 58*, 865–870.
51. Thompson, W. L., & Thompson, T. L., II. (1984). Treating depression in asthmatic patients. *Psychosomatics, 25*, 809–812.
52. Thompson, W. L., & Thompson, T. L., II. (1985). Use of medications in patients with chronic respiratory disease. *Advances in Psychosom Med, 14*, 136–148.
53. Min, S. K. (2006). *New Psychiatry*. Ilchokak.
54. Goodnick, P. J., Henry, J. H., & Buki, V. M. V. (1995). Treatment of depression in patients with diabetes mellitus. *The Journal of Clinical Psychiatry, 56*, 128–136.
55. Kaplan, S. M., Mass, J. W., & Pixley, J. M. (1960). Use of imipramine in diabetics. *JAMA, 174*, 511–517.
56. Unger, J., & Schwartz, Z. (2013). *Diabetes management in primary care* (2nd ed.). Lippincott Williams & Wilkins.
57. Lustman, P. J., & Clouse, R. E. (2005). Depression in diabetic patients: The relationship between mood and glycemic control. *Journal of Diabetes and its Complications, 19*, 113–122.
58. Clayton, A. H., Pradko, J. F., Croft, H. A., et al. (2002). Prevalence of sexual dysfunction among newer antidepressants. *The Journal of Clinical Psychiatry, 63*, 357–366.
59. Deshmukh, R., & Franco, K. (2003). Managing weight gain as a side effect of antidepressant therapy. *Cleveland Clinic Journal of Medicine, 70*, 614–623.
60. Nelson, J. C. (1997). Safety and tolerability of the new antidepressants. *The Journal of Clinical Psychiatry, 58*(Suppl 6), 26–31.

61. Settle, E. C., Jr. (1992). Antidepressant side effects: Issues and options. *The Journal of Clinical Psychiatry, 10*, 48–61.
62. Teicher, M. H., Cohen, B. M., & Baldessarini, R. J. (1988). Severe daytime somnolence in patients treated with an MAOI. *The American Journal of Psychiatry, 145*, 1552–1556.
63. Kunik, M. E., Veazey, C., Cully, J. A., et al. (2008). COPD education and cognitive behavioral therapy group treatment for clinically significant symptoms of depression and anxiety in COPD patients: A randomized controlled trial. *Psychological Medicine, 38*, 3853–3896.
64. Smith, S. M., Sonego, S., Ketcheson, L., et al. (2014). A review of the effectiveness of psychological interventions used for anxiety and depression in chronic obstructive pulmonary disease. *BMJ Open Respiratory Research, 1*, e000042.
65. Sirey, J. A., Raue, P. J., & Alexopoulos, G. S. (2007). An intervention to improve depression care in older adults with COPD. *International Journal of Geriatric Psychiatry, 22*, 154–159.
66. Coventry, P. A., Bower, P., Keyworth, C., et al. (2013). The effect of complex interventions on depression and anxiety in chronic obstructive pulmonary disease: Systematic review and meta-analysis. *PLoS One, 8*, e60532.
67. Rackley, S., & Bostwick, J. M. (2012). Depression in medically ill patients. *The Psychiatric Clinics of North America, 35*, 231–247.

Chapter 13
Anxiety in the Medically Ill

13.1 Sources of Anxiety in Medical Patients

An effective approach for medical patients with anxiety needs to address three sequential dimensions as follows [1]:

1. The clinician should look for the possibility of an underlying medical basis for the anxiety.
2. A past history should be obtained to determine if the patient's anxiety is part of an underlying psychiatric disorder.
3. It should be assessed whether anxiety represents a psychologic response to a physical illness.

13.1.1 Physical Diseases and Substances Presenting as Anxiety

Physical diseases that can present with anxiety as a prominent symptom (anxiety disorder due to another medical condition in the DSM-5) include neurological (e.g., complex partial seizures, post-concussion syndrome, acute neurological injury), cardiovascular (e.g., angina pectoris, cardiac arrhythmias), respiratory (e.g., hyperventilation syndrome, bronchial asthma, chronic obstructive pulmonary disease (COPD), recurrent pulmonary embolism), endocrine (e.g., hyperthyroidism, hypoparathyroidism/hyperparathyroidism), and metabolic diseases (e.g., hypoglycemia) [1, 2]. Pheochromocytoma, Cushing's syndrome, hypomagnesemia, hyponatremia, renal failure, and other electrolyte imbalances may also be associated with anxiety [3–7].

Substance-induced anxiety disorders (substance/medication-induced anxiety disorder in the DSM-5) include intoxication with caffeine, cocaine, amphetamine, and neuroleptics, and withdrawal from alcohol, nicotine, sedative-hypnotics, and

K. B. Koh, *Body, Mind and Spirituality*, https://doi.org/10.1007/978-3-032-11214-9_13

narcotics [2]. In addition, α-adrenergic stimulants (e.g., phenylpropanolamine, ephedrine), bronchodilators (e.g., isoproterenol, epinephrine, theophylline), calcium channel blockers (e.g., verapamil, nifedipine, diltiazem), and antihistamines have been reported to cause anxiety [8–13].

13.1.2 Concurrent Psychiatric Disorders in Medical Patients

The second step in evaluating the presentation of anxiety in a medical patient is to evaluate the possibility of underlying psychiatric disorders such as generalized anxiety disorder, panic disorder, somatic symptoms and related disorders, mood disorders, and borderline personality disorder [1].

13.1.3 Psychosocial Anxiety in Medical Patients

No evaluation of the anxious medical patient is complete without an inquiry into the psychosocial dimensions of the patient's experience. Potential psychological sources of anxiety include isolation, dependency (loss of independence), loss of bodily integrity, and dying. For example, a sense of panic may occur in patients receiving chronic dialysis who cannot tolerate dependence on the machine [1].

Misinterpretations of Physical Sensations

According to the cognitive model, panic attacks occur when catastrophic misinterpretations of ambiguous physical sensations (e.g., shortness of breath, increased heart rate) increase arousal. Similarly, dyspnea in patients with COPD is open to catastrophic misinterpretation [14].

In addition, noncardiac chest pain (e.g., gastroesophageal reflux) can be misinterpreted as a serious cardiac disease that causes anxiety [15].

13.1.4 Anxiety in the Intensive Care Setting

Patients with myocardial infarction may experience fear of death or disability and anxiety related to the restriction of their ability to perform daily activities, which may be associated with feelings of helplessness and loss of control [16–18]. In these patients, transfer from the cardiac care unit (CCU) to a general medical ward is often accompanied by a marked increase in anxiety, which is attributed to the loss of constant supervision and intensive monitoring [19].

13.2 Evaluation for Differential Diagnosis

When anxiety symptoms occur in patients with a medical illness, a psychiatrist's ability to rapidly identify anxiety and make a proper differential diagnosis is important because it can save lives. For example, a patient with deteriorating cardiac or pulmonary function may be misidentified as primarily "anxious" and referred to the psychiatrist. Changes in the patient's medical status are missed until the situation becomes critical [20].

When acute anxiety is encountered, clinicians must rule out a rapidly worsening medical condition, substance-induced anxiety (toxicity or withdrawal), and a psychological reaction to stressors or fear associated with the medical illness [20, 21].

During evaluation of medically ill individuals with chronic anxiety, clinicians must rule out medical disorders that mimic anxiety disorders, psychiatric disorders associated with anxiety symptoms, and poor adjustment to medical illness [21].

The clinician should also know whether the medical condition and the anxiety symptoms have been closely related in the literature [2].

Even for apparently healthy patients, particular scrutiny should be paid to more common conditions associated with anxiety, such as arrhythmias, thyroid abnormalities, excessive caffeine intake, and the use of other drugs. Additionally, withdrawal from medications or substances of abuse should be considered. Anxiety-like symptoms may be the first clue to withdrawal syndrome in a patient with unreported regular sedative-hypnotic (e.g., benzodiazepine) or alcohol use [22].

13.3 Management

The management of physical disease-induced anxiety should be preceded by the treatment of the physical disease [23]. The primary treatment of substance-induced anxiety disorder is the removal of the causally involved substance. When anxiety disorder symptoms are present for a significant period after the physical disease has been treated or the substance use has stopped, treatment of the anxiety disorder symptoms with psychopharmacotherapy or psychotherapy or both may be appropriate. Behavioral therapy can also be used efficiently [2].

Cognitive behavior therapy (CBT), based on the cognitive model of panic, is known to be useful for addressing panic attacks in medically ill patients, especially in patients with COPD. Therefore, mental health professionals should collaborate with multidisciplinary medical teams to prevent and treat panic attacks and panic disorder in these patients [14].

13.3.1 Psychopharmacological Management

Psychopharmacotherapy, such as the use of benzodiazepines and antidepressants (e.g., selective serotonin reuptake inhibitors (SSRIs)), may help decrease anxiety symptoms in medically ill patients [2, 24]. However, nonbenzodiazepine antianxiety agents, such as buspirone, may be preferable to benzodiazepines in some cases. Buspirone notably has lesser sedative effects than benzodiazepines [25, 26].

Benzodiazepines

Benzodiazepines can be categorized into long- (e.g., diazepam) and short-acting (e.g., lorazepam) classes. Repeated use of long-acting benzodiazepines may lead to the accumulation and potential impairment of cognitive and motor performance. Such drug accumulation is a special risk to consider with long-acting benzodiazepines, especially in older patients and those with liver impairment [27, 28].

The most common adverse effects of benzodiazepines involve central nervous system (CNS) depression, such as muscle weakness, ataxia, dysarthria, vertigo, somnolence, and confusion [1]. Benzodiazepines may also be associated with amnesia [29].

Benzodiazepine withdrawal symptoms include anxiety, insomnia, dizziness, headache, anorexia, hypotension, hyperthermia, and neuromuscular irritability. Withdrawal symptoms can be minimized by tapering the dose. During withdrawal, autonomic symptoms can be relieved by a β-adrenergic blocker such as propranolol [29].

Clinically, benzodiazepines are not used only to treat anxiety. For example, alprazolam is mainly used as an antianxiety agent, triazolam as a hypnotic, and clonazepam as an anticonvulsant. Clonazepam is also helpful for relieving anxiety in patients with obsessive-compulsive disorder [30].

The dosages and half-lives of antianxiety agents are shown in Table 13.1 [31].

Buspirone

Buspirone is a nonbenzodiazepine antianxiety agent. Unlike benzodiazepines, buspirone does not act as a muscle relaxant or anticonvulsant, or impact hypnotic activity [25, 26]. Major side effects include dizziness, headaches, and nervousness. Though withdrawal syndrome has not been reported, it is important to be aware that the anxiolytic effects of buspirone may take several weeks to occur [1]. Therefore, this drug may be useful for the chronic treatment of anxiety.

Table 13.1 The dosages and half-lives of antianxiety agents

	Daily dosage (mg)	Half-life (hour)
Benzodiazepine anxiolytics		
Chlordiazepoxide (Librium)	5 ~ 100	12 ~ 48
Diazepam (Valium)	2 ~ 40	20 ~ 90
Ethyl loflazepate (Victan)	1 ~ 4	77 (average)
Lorazepam (Ativan)	1 ~ 4	10 ~ 20
Clonazepam (Rivotril)	0.5 ~ 5.0	18 ~ 28
Alprazolam (Xanax)	0.25 ~ 5.0	12 ~ 19
Triazolam (Halcion)	0.125 ~ 0.25	2.5 ~ 3.5
Nonbenzodiazepine anxiolytics		
Buspirone (Buspar)	15 ~ 60	2 ~ 3
β-Adrenergic blocker		
Propranolol (indenol)	20 ~ 160	3 ~ 6

Propranolol

Propranolol, a β-adrenergic blocker, can antagonize peripheral autonomic symptoms of anxiety such as tachycardia and tremor. In addition, this drug is helpful in relieving nervousness, restlessness, and tension [32]. The most common side effects include depression and weakness. Contraindications to the use of β-blockers include bradycardia, atrioventricular block, congestive heart failure, and COPD [1].

Antidepressants

Antidepressants are known to be effective in the treatment of anxiety. Tricyclics, such as amitriptyline, have been recommended for the treatment of panic attacks [33, 34] and may be effective in the treatment of chronic anxiety [35]. In addition, SSRIs are known to protect against anxiety associated with phobia, panic reactions, and obsessive-compulsive symptoms [30].

13.3.2 Psychosocial Treatment

Psychosocial treatment includes psychotherapy, behavioral therapy, and family interventions. These methods provide accurate medical information (e.g., diagnosis and prognosis), explain the role and meaning of the monitoring equipment, provide emotional support and reassurance, and reinforce the appropriate use of denial [36–39]. Providing patients with information about their illness may shorten their hospital stays [40].

Psychotherapy

Psychotherapy, particularly CBT, helps reduce anxiety in medically ill patients [41]. The interviewer's attitude must convey a sense of interest in understanding what concerns the patient [1]. In addition to separation and loss, real and symbolic physical threats are common themes explored in an initial interview [42].

Sharing information about the illness and diagnosis should be considered an important means of allowing patients to resume control and may reduce anxiety. Maintenance of regular contact and communication of concerns are valuable positive interventions [1].

With a cognitive approach, patients with severe anxiety or panic attacks can be helped to systematically assess the reality of their worries and to view panic as a catastrophic misinterpretation of otherwise benign bodily sensations [42]. Brief cognitive psychotherapy may also help reduce anxiety, medical complications, and functional disabilities, and hospital stays at follow-up [43].

Behavioral Therapy

Behavioral therapy is usually limited to relaxation training for anxious patients; however, treatment for phobic patients can be initiated in the hospital with desensitization and exposure techniques, depending on the phobic stimulus [42]. Teaching patients relaxation techniques that they may use as needed may also be an effective strategy to reduce anxiety and enhance self-control and self-efficiency [19].

Meditation induces a physiological state of restful alertness [44].

Family Interventions

Family interventions may prove therapeutically expedient because disrupted relationships with family members may be provocative [42].

Case

A 58-year-old male patient visited the department of psychiatry as an outpatient with several bouts of chest tightness, dizziness, sensation of impending death, and anxiety. His blood pressure was 180/140 mmHg, and he was diagnosed with panic disorder comorbid with essential hypertension.

Through a series of interviews, it became obvious that his personality was obsessive-compulsive. He always had to put all his clothes and socks in the same places and felt relieved only when the toilet roll was hung in the correct direction. He also felt uncomfortable on days he skipped his exercise, even if it happened only once. His blood pressure was generally high, probably because of his being constantly tense. He used to take his blood pressure several times a day and showed sensitive responses to changes in blood pressure. Atenolol (Tenormin) 50 mg, an antihypertensive drug, was given once a day and ethyl loflazepate 1 mg, an antianxiety agent, was given twice a day. He was recommended to do muscle relaxation to relieve tension and anxiety. He was also asked to think and act unlike the way he used to do. He started to challenge his obsessive thinking and compulsive behavior, saying "so what if I take off my socks anywhere?" and "so what if I skip exercise one day?" From that time onwards, he felt less anxious and tense.

He did not experience fear of impending death anymore, even though he still felt somewhat anxious. In addition, he was not anxious anymore when he did not take his blood pressure, and thus decided not to take it anymore. Moreover, he realized that his personality changed markedly, from being rigid and inflexible to being able to listen to others, saying to himself "am I that great?" His anxiety was significantly reduced and his blood pressure remained within the normal range. Eventually, ethyl loflazepate was discontinued, and the patient stayed symptom-free with only Tenormin 25 mg once a day.

13.4 Summary

1. Clinicians should know whether a medical condition or substance has been closely associated with anxiety symptoms in the literature.
2. Assessment of anxiety in medically ill patients requires the examination of biological and psychosocial factors.
3. Clinicians should address major psychological issues such as isolation, dependency, loss of bodily integrity, and dying, which are commonly associated with anxiety in medically ill patients.
4. Management of physical disease-induced anxiety should be preceded by the treatment of physical diseases.
5. The primary treatment of substance-induced anxiety disorder is the removal of the causally involved substance.
6. Any successful intervention for these patients should involve a biopsychosocial approach that includes psychopharmacological and psychosocial treatment.
7. Cognitive behavioral therapy can be used to treat panic attacks in medically ill patients.

References

1. Goldberg, R. J. (1987). Anxiety in the medically ill. In A. Stoudemire & B. S. Fogel (Eds.), *Principles of medical psychiatry*. Grune & Stratton Inc.
2. Sadock, B. J., & Sadock, V. A. (2003). *Synopsis of psychiatry—Behavioral sciences/clinical psychiatry* (pp. 636–642). Lippincott Williams & Wilkins.
3. Lishman, W. A. (1978). *Organic psychiatry (endocrine disorders and metabolic disorders)*. Blackwell.

4. Hall, R. C. W., & Joffe, J. R. (1973). Hypomagnesemia: Physical and psychiatric symptoms. *JAMA, 224*, 1749–1751.
5. Gehi, M. M., Rosenthal, R. H., Fizette, N. B., et al. (1981). Psychiatric manifestations of hyponatremia. *Psychosomatics, 22*, 739–743.
6. Marshall, J. R. (1979). Neuropsychiatric aspects of renal failure. *The Journal of Clinical Psychiatry, 40*, 81–85.
7. Webb, W. L., & Gehi, M. (1981). Electrolyte and fluid imbalance: Neuropsychiatric manifestations. *Psychosomatics, 22*, 199–203.
8. Jacobs, M. A., Senior, R. M., & Kessler, G. (1976). Clinical experience with theophylline: Relationship between dosage, serum concentration, and toxicity. *JAMA, 235*, 1983–1986.
9. Bela, S. V., & Raftery, E. V. (1980). The role of verapamil in chronic stable angina: A controlled study with computerized multistage treadmill exercise. *Lancet, 1*, 841–844.
10. Mueller, H. S., & Chahine, R. A. (1981). Interim report of multicenter double-blind placebo-controlled studies of nifedipine in chronic stable angina. *The American Journal of Medicine, 71*, 645–657.
11. Rickenberger, R. L., Psytowsky, E. N., Heger, J. J., et al. (1980). Effects of intravenous and chronic oral verapamil administration in patients with supraventricular arrhythmias. *Circulation, 62*, 996–1010.
12. Singh, B. N., Elklrodt, G., & Peter, C. T. (1978). Verapamil: A review of its pharmacological properties and therapeutic use. *Drugs, 15*, 169–197.
13. Abramowicz, M. (1984). Drugs that cause psychiatric symptoms. *Med Letter, 26*, 75–78.
14. Livermore N1, Sharpe L, McKenzie D. (2010). Panic attacks and panic disorder in chronic obstructive pulmonary disease: A cognitive behavioral perspective. *Respiratory Medicine, 104*, 1246–1253.
15. Ketterer, M. W. (1999). Cognitive/behavioral therapy of anxiety in the medically ill: Cardiac settings. *Seminars in Clinical Neuropsychiatry, 4*, 148–153.
16. Cassem, N. H., & Hackett, T. P. (1971). Psychiatric consultation in a coronary care unit. *Annals of Internal Medicine, 75*, 9–14.
17. Krantz, D. S. (1980). Cognitive process and recovery from heart attack: A review and theoretical analysis. *Journal of Human Stress, 6*, 27–38.
18. Stern, T. A. (1985). The management of depression and anxiety following myocardial infarction. *Mount Sinai Journal of Medicine, 52*, 623–633.
19. Goldstein, M. G. (1987). Intensive care unit syndromes. In A. Stoudemire & B. S. Fogel (Eds.), *Principles of medical psychiatry* (pp. 403–421). Grune & Stratton Inc.
20. Wise, M. G., & Rieck, S. O. (1993). Diagnostic considerations and treatment approaches to underlying anxiety in the medically ill. *The Journal of Clinical Psychiatry, 54*(Suppl), 22–26.
21. Wise, M. G., & Griffies, W. S. (1995). A combined treatment approach to anxiety in the medically ill. *The Journal of Clinical Psychiatry, 56*(Suppl 2), 14–19.
22. Avant, R. F. (1983). Diagnosis and management of depression in the office setting. *Fam Pract Res, 5*(Suppl 1), 41.
23. Bernstein, J. G. (1995). *Handbook of drug therapy in psychiatry*. Mosby.
24. Mago, R., Gomez, J. P., Gupta, N., et al. (2006). Anxiety in medically ill patients. *Current Psychiatry Reports, 8*, 228–233.
25. Cohn, J. B., & Wilcox, C. S. (1986). Low-sedation potential of buspirone compared with alprazolam and lorazepam in the treatment of anxious patients: A double-blind study. *The Journal of Clinical Psychiatry, 47*, 409–412.
26. Newton, R. E., Marunycz, J. D., Alderdice, M. T., et al. (1986). Review of the side-effect profile of buspirone. *The American Journal of Medicine, 80*(Suppl 3B), 17–21.
27. Greenblatt, D. J., Allen, M. D., Harmatz, M. J., et al. (1980). *Diazepam disposition determinants. Clin Pharamcol Ther, 27*, 301–312.
28. Hoyumpa, A. M. (1978). Disposition and elimination of minor tranquilizers in the aged and in patients with liver disease. *Southern Med J, 71*, 23–28.
29. Abernethy, D. R., Greenblatt, D. J., & Shader, R. I. (1981). Treatment of diazepam withdrawal syndrome with propranolol. *Annals of Internal Medicine, 94*, 354–355.

30. Jimerson, D. C., & Docherty, J. P. (1986). *Psychopharmacology consultation.* Am Psychiatric Press Inc.
31. Koh, K. B. (2018). *Stress and somatic symptoms: Biopsychosociospiritual perspectives.* Springer.
32. Kathol, R. G., Noyes, R., Jr., Slymen, D. J., et al. (1980). Propranolol in chronic anxiety disorders: A controlled study. *Archives of General Psychiatry, 37*, 1361–1365.
33. Klein, D. F. (1982). Medication in the treatment of panic attacks and phobic states. *Psychopharmacology Bulletin, 18*, 85–90.
34. Pohl, R., Berchou, R., & Rainey, J. M. (1982). Tricyclic antidepressants and monoamine oxidase inhibitors in the treatment of agpraphobia. *Journal of Clinical Psychopharmacology, 2*, 399–407.
35. Lipman, R. S., Covi, L., Downing, R. W., et al. (1981). Pharmacotherapy of anxiety and depression. *Psychopharmacology Bulletin, 17*, 91–103.
36. Thomas SA, Sappington E, Gross HS. Denial in coronary care patients—an objective reassessment. Heart and Lung 1983;12:74–80.
37. Cohen-Cole, S. A. (1985). Interviewing the cardiac patient: I. A practical guide assessing quality of life. *Quality of Life in Cardiovascular Care, 2*, 7–12.
38. Cohen-Cole, S. A., & Bird, J. (1986). Interviewing the cardiac patient: II. A practical guide for helping patients cope with their emotions. *Quality of Life in Cardiovascular Care, 2*, 53–65.
39. Munford, E., Schlessinger, H. J., & Glass, G. V. (1982). The effects of psychological intervention on recovery from surgery and heart attacks: An analysis of the literature. *American Journal of Public Health, 72*, 141–152.
40. Cromwell RL, Butterfield EC, Brayfield FM. Acute myocardial infarction:Reaction and recovery. : Mosby; 1977.
41. Shaffer, K. M., Jacobs, J. M., Coleman, J. N., et al. (2017). Anxiety and depressive symptoms among two seriously medically ill populations and their family caregivers: A comparison and clinical implications. *Neurocritical Care, 27*, 180–186.
42. Rosenbaum, J. F., & Pollack, M. H. (1991). Anxiety. In N. H. Cassem (Ed.), *MGH handbook of general hospital psychiatry* (3rd ed.). Mosby Year Book.
43. Gruen, W. (1975). Effects of brief psychotherapy during the hospitalization period on the recovery process in heart attacks. *J Clin Consult Psychol, 43*, 232–233.
44. Walace RK. Physiological effects of transcendental meditation. Science 1970;e167:1751–4.

Chapter 14
Functional Dyspepsia

14.1 What is Functional Dyspepsia?

Functional dyspepsia (FD) is a clinical syndrome characterized by chronic early satiety, postprandial fullness, and epigastric pain or burning [1]. It can be subdivided into postprandial distress syndrome (comprising early satiety and/or postprandial fullness) and epigastric pain syndrome [2].

Functional dyspepsia is a heterogeneous condition with multiple causes [3–5]. In some cases, the gastric acid associated with gastroesophageal reflux may play a significant role in FD, whereas in others, abnormal motility, infection, stressful life events, and personality may play a more important role.

14.2 Psychosocial Factors

The psychosocial factors associated with the onset or aggravation of FD include negative emotions such as anxiety or depression, stress, personality, coping strategies, and lifestyle. Among these, life stress is a major psychological factor associated with FD. Severe life stressors, especially the disruption of close relationships, precede the onset of functional abdominal pain significantly more often than the onset of organic abdominal illness [6].

Alexithymia (i.e., difficulty in verbally expressing emotions) is also considered an etiological factor of FD [7]. Patients with FD tend to show somatothymia, that is, the tendency to communicate their psychological distress through somatic symptoms. This tendency is particularly prominent in patients from a low socioeconomic status [8].

Therefore, it is crucial for physicians to consider psychological factors when evaluating patients with FD.

K. B. Koh, *Body, Mind and Spirituality*, https://doi.org/10.1007/978-3-032-11214-9_14

Case 1
A 60-year-old female patient visited the department of psychiatry because of persistent abdominal discomfort and pain, despite no abnormalities found on gastroendoscopic examination. Accompanied by her elder sister, she looked exhausted, but denied any psychological stressor. Her symptoms were considerably improved after a 4-week-long administration of sertraline, an antidepressant, and ethyl loflazepate, an antianxiety agent. Thereafter, she began to complain of her symptoms again with a grimacing face. At that time, she expressed her conflict with her daughter-in-law, saying "She did not visit me during the period of Chuseok (Korean Thanksgiving Day). She also avoided seeing me even when she visited my neighbor. I do not know how to deal with this."

Case 2
A 50-year-old female patient was admitted to the department of internal medicine because of abdominal pain, nausea, and vomiting, but laboratory findings showed no abnormalities. She was thus referred and then transferred to the department of psychiatry. Her symptoms were exacerbated whenever she visited her sister-in-law and got back home. Later, she said, "she bought a lot of land with the money we had lent her, and later the price of the land jumped and she got rich. However, she did not thank me at all." She felt very disappointed at her sister-in-law's cold attitude.

As seen in these cases, patients with functional dyspepsia often show resistance to expressing their own conflicts or stressful situations at first. Over time, however, or by using a therapeutic technique such as cognitive behavioral therapy, their stressful situations can be elicited from them.

Expression of Their Conflictful Situations Itself Might Be an Important Therapeutic Gate or a Signal of Relief of Symptoms in Such Patients.

14.3 Treatment

14.3.1 Psychotherapy

If physicians are certain that there are no organic diseases, they should avoid conducting examinations and explain why the patient is in discomfort. Physicians' reassurance (e.g., "There are no abnormalities in their endoscopic findings" and "You have no severe diseases at all") is not only therapeutically effective but also plays an important role in reducing repetitive medical examinations in patients with chronic symptoms [9]. In addition, changes in lifestyle, such as avoiding alcohol and coffee consumption and reducing body weight, are needed for treating FD [10].

Cognitive behavioral therapy (CBT), which includes cognitive therapy and muscle relaxation, can be used for patients with FD [11]. Therapists' explanations for symptoms may help patients recognize the situations that elicit pain as well as the outcome of pain [12].

Formal psychotherapy is recommended for patients with persistent symptoms [11]. However, CBT can be attempted in cases in which persistent symptoms are related to the patients' abnormal beliefs about health or preoccupation with somatic symptoms, as is often seen in patients with somatic symptom disorder and hypochondriasis [13, 14]. In particular, CBT can be suitable for symptoms of uncertain etiology because the self-assessment and behavioral components of the therapy can help identify their causes and improve the symptoms [15].

14.3.2 Biological Treatment

General Pharmacotherapy

In patients with mild FD symptoms, reassurance and lifestyle adjustments are often sufficient. However, for patients with severe or persistent symptoms, it is desirable to use proton pump inhibitors (PPIs), prokinetics, and psychotropic agents. Eradication is recommended for patients with Helicobacter pylori infection. For epigastric pain syndrome, PPIs (e.g., omeprazole) are the initial therapy of choice, whereas prokinetics (e.g., mosapride and acotiamide) are preferred for postprandial distress syndrome [2].

Psychopharmacotherapy

Antianxiety agents such as lorazepam and diazepam are known to be more effective than placebos in treating patients with functional gastrointestinal disorders, including FD [16].

Tricyclic antidepressants such as amitriptyline can be used for FD patients with high levels of depression as they do not seem to stimulate the gastrointestinal system. However, the anticholinergic effects of these drugs can delay gastrointestinal motility. In particular, the use of the antidepressants is considered for refractory symptoms of FD or epigastric pain syndrome [2]. Mirtazapine is recommended for FD patients with weight loss. However, selective serotonin reuptake inhibitors are not preferred for these patients [1, 2].

Drug–Drug Interaction

The combined use of cimetidine and tricyclic antidepressants increases the risk of cumulative drug toxicity (e.g., decreased gastrointestinal motility related to the anticholinergic effects of tricyclic antidepressants). Cimetidine also inhibits the metabolism of venlafaxine [17].

14.4 Summary

1. Explanations for symptoms, reassurance, modification of lifestyles, and cognitive behavioral therapy may help treat patients with functional dyspepsia (FD).
2. A combination of psychotherapy and muscle relaxation helps reduce the onset of pain and relieve FD symptoms.
3. In FD patients with mild symptoms, reassurance and lifestyle adjustments are often sufficient.
4. For those with more severe or persistent symptoms, the use of proton pump inhibitors (PPIs), prokinetics, and psychotropic agents is recommended.
5. Tricyclic antidepressants can be used for refractory symptoms of FD, especially in epigastric pain syndrome.
6. Mirtazapine is recommended for FD patients with weight loss.

References

1. Haug, T. T., Svebak, S., Wilhelmsen, I., et al. (1994). Psychological factors and somatic symptoms in functional dyspepsia: A comparison with duodenal ulcer and healthy controls. *Journal of Psychosomatic Research, 38*, 281–291.
2. Vanheel, H., & Tack, J. (2014). Therapeutic options for functional dyspepsia. *Digestive Diseases, 32*, 230–234.
3. Colin-Jones, D. G. (1988). Management of dyspepsia: Report of a working party. *Lancet, 1*, 576–579.
4. Barsky, A. J., & Klerman, G. L. (1983). Overviews: Hypochondriasis, bodily complaints and somatic styles. *American Journal of Psychiatry, 140*, 273–283.
5. Kellner, R. (1987). Hypochondriasis and somatization. *JAMA, 258*, 2718–2722.
6. Creed, F., Craig, T., & Farmer, R. (1988). Functional abdominal pain, psychiatric illness, and life events. *Gut, 29*, 235–242.
7. Talley, N. J., Ellard, K., Jones, M., et al. (1988). Suppression of emotions in essential dyspepsia and chronic ulcer: A case-control study. *Scandinavian Journal of Gastroenterology, 23*, 337–340.
8. Yates, W. R. (2000). Gastrointestinal disorders. In B. J. Sadock, V. A. Sadock (Eds.), *Comprehensive textbook of psychiatry* (7th ed). Lippincott Williams & Wilkins.
9. Morris, C. (1991). Invited review: Non-ulcer dyspepsia. *Journal of Psychosomatic Research, 35*, 129–140.
10. Langeluddecke, P., Goulston, K., & Tennant, C. (1990). Psychological factors in dyspepsia of unknown cause: A comparison with peptic ulcer disease. *Journal of Psychosomatic Research, 34*, 215–222.
11. Bates, S., Sjoden, P. O., & Nyren, O. (1988). Behavioral treatment of non-ulcer dyspepsia. *Scandinavian Journal of Behaviour Therapy, 17*, 155–165.
12. Piacentino, D., Cantarini, R., Alfonsi, M., et al. (2011). Psychopathological features of irritable bowel syndrome patients with and without functional dyspepsia: A cross sectional study. *BMC Gastroenterology, 11*, 94.
13. Klimes, I., Mayou, R. A., Pearce, M. J., et al. (1990). Psychological treatment for atypical noncardiac chest pain: A controlled evaluation. *Psychological Medicine, 20*, 605–611.
14. Salkovskis, P. M., & Warwick, H. M. (1986). Morbid preoccupations, health anxiety and reassurance: A cognitive-behavioral approach to hypochondriasis. *Behaviour Research and Therapy, 24*, 597–602.

15. Koh, K. B. (2011). *Stress and psychosomatic medicine* (2nd ed., pp. 426–438). Ilchokak.
16. Baume, P., Tracey, M., & Dawson, L. (1975). Efficacy of two minor tranquilizers in relieving symptoms of functional gastrointestinal distress. *Australian and New Zealand Journal of Medicine, 5*, 503–506.
17. Beliles, K., & Stoudemire, A. (1998). Psychopharmacologic treatment of depression in the medically ill. *Psychosomatics, 39*, S2–S19.

Chapter 15
Post-Stroke Depression

15.1 What Is a Stroke?

A stroke is defined as a sudden loss of blood supply to the brain leading to permanent damage caused by thrombotic, embolic, or hemorrhagic events. It is the leading cause of death in patients aged 50 years and above [1].

15.2 Psychological Sequelae of Stroke

The physical and/or psychological sequelae of this disease may be devastating for both the patients and their families. In particular, depression during the illness hinders therapeutic efforts [2].

Post-stroke depression is the most common neuropsychiatric condition after stroke [3–5]. Several factors such as stroke severity, physical disability, and cognitive impairment have been consistently associated with depression following stroke [6]. In particular, the severity of disability is one of the strongest risk factors of post-stroke depression [7].

Grief and demoralization would be expected as normal, but withdrawal associated with hopelessness and refusal to participate in potentially effective rehabilitation efforts would be considered maladaptive [8]. Stoke can also damage the patient's self-esteem [9].

K. B. Koh, *Body, Mind and Spirituality*, https://doi.org/10.1007/978-3-032-11214-9_15

15.3 Management of Post-Stroke Depression

Early and aggressive treatment of post-stroke depression is required to minimize the cognitive and performance deficits that depression inflicts on the patient during the recovery period [9]. The biopsychosocial approach to the treatment of depression is highly recommended because post-stroke depression may result from a combination of biological, psychological, and social factors [2].

The major goals of the treatment regimens for post-stroke depression are to improve mood and quality of life, use healthcare resources appropriately, and reduce the risk of medical complications [10]. The management of post-stroke depression includes psychopharmacotherapy, psychotherapy, and physical exercise.

15.3.1 Psychopharmacotherapy

Antidepressants can be effective in treating moderate and severe depressive disorders, such as major depressive disorder [11]. Sertraline and citalopram have demonstrated significant efficacy as antidepressants [12, 13]. In particular, sertraline, paroxetine, and venlafaxine are preferred because of their relatively short half-life [13]. Therefore, it is advisable to treat post-stroke depression with selective serotonin reuptake inhibitors of proven efficacy and switch to nortriptyline if there is no significant improvement after an adequate trial and there are no contraindications for the use of tricyclics [12].

Antidepressants should be continued at least for 4 months after initial recovery and should be changed if no response is seen after 6 weeks [14]. Antidepressant treatment can then be slowly withdrawn, or in case of relapse, it can be continued for a longer duration [15, 16].

15.3.2 Psychological Interventions

Psychological treatments include behavioral therapy and cognitive behavioral therapy [17]. Treatment of adjustment disorder after a stroke is primarily psychosocial. The focus should be on nonspecific support, education, and clarification of the individual's conflicts in the context of the physical illness [8]. In particular, emphasis should be placed on maintaining the person's self-esteem in psychotherapy [9]. Support from family and friends is also essential in treatment.

Cognitive Behavioral Therapy

Cognitive behavioral therapy (CBT) has a strong and positive effect on post-stroke depression because it builds confidence and improves the individual's daily lifestyle through several activities. It is designed to challenge dysfunctional thoughts or beliefs associated with low mood and to collaboratively establish more functional thoughts or beliefs [18]. Particularly, CBT is based on providing insights using psychoeducation, collaborative empiricism, and active problem-solving; assessing the quality of support; and improving the patient's adaptation to a new lifestyle after a stroke [19]. However, patients with cognitive impairment and/or aphasia are not eligible for this form of treatment [11].

In general, approximately six to eight regular sessions should be provided to patients over a period of 10–12 weeks, with most people experiencing improvements in mood and/or a reduction in symptoms after 2 months of therapy. Responses to therapy should be reviewed after eight sessions. A therapy extension period of 6 months is considered necessary for a person who has multiple issues or severe comorbidity [6].

In some studies, CBT has failed to provide evidence of its effectiveness in treating post-stroke depression [20, 21].

Given these contradictory results, psychotherapy should be combined with antidepressants to reduce residual symptoms and the risk of relapse in patients with severe depression and in those with moderate or severe depression who refuse antidepressants [22].

Physical Exercise, Activity, Physical, and Speech Therapy

Physical exercise during the subacute recovery phase of stroke has a beneficial effect on depressive symptoms [23]. In most psychological treatments, behavioral activation is often involved, which addresses the problem of limitations in activity. Some of these approaches primarily focus on the meaningfulness of the activity during the treatment, which may help intensify and maintain cognition and target depression [24]. Additionally, physical therapy and speech therapy may also be helpful for patients with post-stroke depression in regaining a sense of sound body and self-esteem.

15.3.3 Integrated Care

Multidisciplinary and integrative approaches are recommended for assessing and treating post-stroke depression [15, 25]. Thus, the treatment of depression after stroke should include psychiatrists or psychologists, neurologists or neurosurgeons, rehabilitation medicine specialists, nurses, physical therapists, and speech therapists. Integrative approaches include screening for depression and assessing the severity of depression using psychological instruments such as the Beck Depression Inventory II and Hamilton Rating Scale for Depression. Psychiatric consultations and psychopharmacotherapy are also needed to assess and treat depression in these patients [26].

Case 1

A 49-year-old female patient was admitted to the department of neurosurgery via the emergency room with a sudden onset of headache and loss of consciousness. She underwent surgery with the diagnosis of aneurysmal rupture at the middle cerebral artery. However, she suffered from its sequelae, including right hemiparesis, aphasia, impaired orientation to time, memory disturbance, and diminished intellectual functioning. She was then transferred to the department of rehabilitation medicine, where she underwent physical therapy and speech therapy. She was referred to the department of psychiatry after being discharged from the hospital.

On her first visit to the outpatient psychiatry department, a mental status examination revealed signs of an organic mental disorder and of an adjustment disorder with depression: weeping spells, loss of self-esteem caused by loss of bodily functions, impaired memory, and slurred speech. She received supportive psychotherapy and medication including haloperidol and fluoxetine biweekly for 3 months and then monthly for 2 years. Additionally, she underwent physical therapy and speech therapy at the department of rehabilitation medicine. Despite her many disabilities, she continued to practice writing and speaking briefly.

Physical therapy helped her lift her right hand to some degree, but not completely. It was possible for the patient to communicate with her family members and friends with the help of the speech therapist, but it was still difficult for her to form sentences. She was sometimes frustrated by her limited ability to speak and lift her arm, but she looked joyful as her slurred speech improved. She continued to exercise outside her house and to receive physical therapy at home everyday.

About five months later, she reported feeling thankful for her husband's warm and encouraging attitude. Her speech had drastically improved, and she was able to talk with her friends on the phone, albeit fast. She was surprised that she was again able to say numbers in German as she had forgotten how to immediately after her illness. Her memory also improved. However, she still exhibited bouts of sudden tearfulness, particularly when recalling her survival from her near-death experience. She began to write letters to her friends and her two sons who had been studying abroad. She was able to recall the names of her friends completely. Her stuttering also notably improved. Her friends encouraged her by saying, "Now you can talk better than one month ago" and "You do not stutter at all," although she did not notice those changes.

She continued to exercise at the fitness center. She was able to go outside without being accompanied by her husband. She began to understand the Chinese characters she had forgotten after her illness. Additionally, her vocabulary use and understanding increased. She was also able to speak in a low tone and was surprised that she was still able to completely lift her right arm.

Case 2

A 70-year-old male patient with stroke was admitted to the department of neurology. His brain lesion was found to have multiple diffuse embolisms, the prognosis of which was judged to be irreversible and hopeless by the neurologist. The patient was transferred to the department of rehabilitation medicine for supportive care of the stroke sequelae, including hemiparesis and aphasia. He required physical therapy and speech therapy, but declined treatment and refused to eat.

He was referred to the department of psychiatry for consultation. He was severely depressed because he could no longer live as an independent person and instead had to be absolutely dependent on his wife. He was diagnosed with major depressive disorder and an antidepressant, sertraline (Zoloft), was administered. His wife, who had devoted most of her time to taking care of him, was also tearful and appeared tired because of her husband's pessimistic and uncooperative attitude. After four weeks of treatment with the antidepressant, his depression was greatly improved. Thereafter, he began to participate in physical therapy and speech therapy. Even after being discharged from the hospital, he continued to exercise and to receive physical therapy and speech therapy. They moved to Canada where their daughter was living. After seven years, he returned to Korea with his wife and was assessed at the hospital. He was observed to be able to put on his shoes, stand up, and walk with the help of his wife, and even talk, which was very surprising given his status at the last visit.

These two cases show the impact that stroke sequelae have on patients' and their partners' emotions and self-esteem. This suggests that a multidisciplinary approach could be effective in assessing and treating post-stroke depression. In particular, treatment of post-stroke depression should be integrative, including biological treatment such as antidepressants, psychotherapy, physical exercise, and physical and speech therapy [27].

15.4 Summary

1. The physical and/or psychological sequelae of stroke may be devastating for both the patients and their families.
2. Depression during this illness hinders therapeutic efforts.
3. It is advisable to treat post-stroke depression with selective serotonin reuptake inhibitors of proven efficacy.
4. Multidisciplinary and integrative approaches are recommended for assessing and treating post-stroke depression.

References

1. Robinson, R. G., & Spalletta, G. (2010). Poststroke depression: A review. *Canadian Journal of Psychiatry, 55*, 341–349.

2. Whyte, E. M., & Mulsant, B. H. (2002). Post-stroke depression: Epidemiology, pathophysiology, and biological treatment. *Biological Psychiatry, 52*, 253–264.
3. Robinson, R. G. (1997). Neuropsychiatric consequences of stroke. *Annual Review of Medicine, 48*, 217–229.
4. Wolfe, C. D. A. (2000). The impact of stroke. *British Medical Bulletin, 56*, 275–286.
5. Williams, L. S., Ghose, S. S., & Swindle, R. W. (2004). Depression and other mental health diagnoses increase mortality risk after ischemic stroke. *American Journal of Psychiatry, 161*, 1090–1095.
6. Hackett, M., & Anderson, C. (2005). Treatment options for post-stroke depression in the elderly. *Aging and Health, 1*, 95–105.
7. Murphy, E. (1982). Social origins of depression in old age. *British Journal of Psychiatry, 141*, 134–142.
8. Cohen-Cole, S. A., Harpe, C. (1987). Assessment of depression in the medically ill. In A. Stoudemire, & B. S. Fogel, (Eds), *Principles of medical psychiatry*. Grune & Stratton.
9. Cassem, N. H. (1991). Depression. In N. H. Cassem, (Ed.) *MGH handbook of general hospital psychiatry*. Mosby-Year Book.
10. Alexopoulos, G., Buckwalter, K., Olin, J., et al. (2002). Comorbidity of late life depression: An opportunity for research on mechanisms and treatment. *Biological Psychiatry, 52*, 543–558.
11. Lokk, J., & Delbari, A. (2010). Management of depression in elderly stroke patients. *Neuropsychiatric Disease and Treatment, 6*, 539–549.
12. Starkstein, S. E., Mizrahi, R., & Power, B. D. (2008). Antidepressant therapy in post-stroke depression. *Expert Opinion on Pharmacotherapy, 9*, 1291–1298.
13. Cunningham, L. A. (1994). Depression in the medically ill: Choosing an antidepressant. *The Journal of Clinical Psychiatry, 55*, Suppl AJ, 90–7.
14. Snow, V., Lascher, S., & Mottur-Pilson, C. (2000). Pharmacologic treatment of acute major depression and dysthymia: Clinical guideline, part 1. *Annals of Internal Medicine, 132*, 738–742.
15. Turner-stokes, L., Hassan, N. (2002). Depression after stroke: A review of the evidence base to inform the development of an integrated pathway. Part 1: Diagnosis, frequency and impact. *Clinical Rehabilitation, 16*, 231–47.
16. Williams, L. S. (2005). Depression and stroke: Cause or consequence? *Seminars in Neurology, 25*, 396–409.
17. Scogin, F., Welsh, D., Hanson, A., et al. (2006). Evidence-based psychotherapies for depression in older adults. *Clinical Psychology: Science and Practice, 12*, 222–237.
18. Laidlaw, K. (2007). Poststroke depression and CBT with older people. In G. -T. Dolores, M. S. Ann, & W. T. Lary (Eds.), *Handbook of behavioral and cognitive therapies with older adults*. New York: Springer.
19. Gallagher-Thompson, D., Steffen, A., Thompson, L., et al. (2008). *Handbook of behavioral and cognitive therapies with older adults*. Springer.
20. Lincoln, N., & Flannaghan, T. (2003). Cognitive behavioral psychotherapy for depression following stroke: A randomized controlled trial. *Stroke, 34*, 111–115.
21. Hackett, M., Anderson, C., & House, A. (2009). Interventions for treating depression after stroke. *Stroke, 40*, e487–e488.
22. Australian, R. (2004). Australian and New Zealand clinical practice guidelines for the treatment of depression. *Australian and New Zealand Journal of Psychiatry, 38*, 389–407.
23. Lai, S. M., Studenski, S., Richards, L., et al. (2006). Therapeutic exercise and depressive symptoms after stroke. *Journal of the American Geriatrics Society, 54*, 240–247.
24. Fiske, A., Wetherell, J., & Gatz, M. (2009). Depression in older adults. *Ann Rev Clin Psychol, 5*, 363–389.
25. Turner-Stokes, L., Hassan, N., et al. (2002). Managing depression in brain injury rehabilitation: The use of an integrated care pathway and preliminary report of response to sertraline. *Clinical Rehabilitation, 16*, 261–268.
26. Beck, A. T., Ward, C. H., Mendelssohn, M. J., et al. (1961). An inventory for measuring depression. *Archives of General Psychiatry, 4*, 561–571.

27. Koh, K. B. (2013). Poststroke depression: Mechanisms and management. In K. B. Koh, (Ed.), *Somatization and psychosomatic symptoms*. Springer.

Chapter 16
Cancer

16.1 What Does it Mean to Live with Cancer?

Although some cancers that had a very poor prognosis several decades ago are currently being cured, cancer remains a disease associated with hopelessness, pain, fear, and death [1]. Medical developments in cancer diagnosis and treatment have dramatically improved survival rates. As a result, professional attention has shifted from issues related to death and dying to the physical, psychological, and behavioral consequences of rigorous treatment regimens [1, 2].

To live with cancer is much more than adapting to the treatments and their various side effects. There are a host of psychosocial issues with which to cope in addition to the threat of mortality. To understand cancer merely as a biological event is to overlook the innumerable biopsychosocial factors that demand strategic coping from patients and their families [3]. Therefore, quality of life and delayed treatment effects have become important issues [1].

16.2 Effective Communication with Cancer Patients

Getting to know cancer patients as persons is essential. As with anyone else, these individuals gain self-respect from feeling that others value them for what they have done and for their personal qualities. Allowing dying individuals to tell their own stories helps build balanced relationships. They want to be treated as real persons and not as dying patients [4].

K. B. Koh, *Body, Mind and Spirituality*, https://doi.org/10.1007/978-3-032-11214-9_16

16.3 Therapeutic Approaches

16.3.1 General Treatment

The therapeutic goal is to not only help the patient adjust to cancer but also utilize mobilized emotions and issues to resolve existing conflicts [5]. In general, the therapeutic approaches used for patients with cancer are a combination of psychotherapeutic, psychopharmacological, and behavioral techniques [1].

Individual therapy utilizes a crisis-intervention approach in which the therapist (1) encourages the patient to express feelings, (2) offers support and optimism, (3) clarifies feelings, (4) interprets thoughts in psychodynamic terms, (5) encourages the patient to act on his or her circumstances, (6) explores the current situation in the context of the past, (7) focuses on specific relevant psychodynamic issues, and (8) limits the duration of therapy [6].

Clarification of the medical condition and related treatments is important. Informed patients have less fear and anxiety, lower levels of stress, and better functioning coping responses [7]. Relaxation techniques help patients with cancer feel that they can exercise control over their bodies as well as relieve pain and anxiety without extra medication [8].

The therapeutic techniques of choice with each patient and family depend on individual needs and the modalities available [5].

16.3.2 Cognitive Behavioral Therapy

Cognitive behavioral therapy (CBT) can be effectively used in patients with cancer. The overall aims of this treatment are to correct coping deficits, reduce distress levels, reclaim personal control, teach problem-solving methods, and improve morale.

CBT appears most useful for those patients identified as poor copers. First, it addresses patients' coping deficits. Second, a short-term educational intervention focusing on the "here and now" enables the clinician and patient to collaborate in promoting the patient's self-control and responsibility for health. A third advantage of this treatment is cost-effectiveness. This kind of treatment offers patients an opportunity to learn a method for coping with problems while continuing to live with cancer [3].

In an approach that focuses on problem-solving, patients are taught to recognize, confront, and solve commonly encountered cancer problems [9, 10]. The intervention comprises four sessions and follows the general principles of short-term psychotherapy.

In the first session, the patient is informed that they will review the common problems faced by many cancer patients and the best and most practical ways to solve them. Ideas for problem-solving are taught, and patients are encouraged to practice these skills with their own problems. Relaxation is presented as a time-out procedure for managing stress [11]. As a way to promote self-management, the patient is given a "homework" assignment for the week which involves daily relaxation training [3].

In the second session, the therapist notes the patient's progress during the relaxation training. The therapist works with the patient to generate possible problem-solving strategies for their particular issues and develop ways to establish priorities among the various possible approaches.

The third session places a heavy focus on problem-solving. At this point, the therapist explores current personal problems with the patient and applies this approach to these problems [3].

During the fourth session, the patient and therapist evaluate the effectiveness of the approach in dealing with problems during the preceding week together. The philosophy behind this cognitive intervention is that problems can be reorganized into manageable proportions [3].

Behavioral techniques include passive relaxation with visual imagery, progressive muscle relaxation, systematic desensitization, and cognitive distraction [12–14]. In addition, exercise interventions may have beneficial effects on health-related quality of life, including physical functioning, role function, social functioning, and fatigue [15].

16.3.3 Family Therapy

Family therapy is essential for cancer patients. The best way to enable family members to become involved in treatment is to point out that patients and their family members need to communicate with each other and provide them with assistance in coping with cancer when they must live with it [2].

Teaching family members how to relax and cope with cancer can help lower their levels of anxiety and stress related to taking care of the patients [5]. As a result, family members of patients with cancer can reduce the expression of negative emotions such as hostility and criticism toward the patients and provide them with more support [16, 17].

16.3.4 Group Psychotherapy

Group psychotherapy for cancer patients is not only efficient in terms of time and financial cost but also highly effective in improving quality of life; reducing psychological distress, anxiety, and depression; improving coping skills; and reducing symptoms such as pain, nausea, and vomiting [18–20]. Group psychotherapy may allow patients with cancer to receive support from others (patients or non-patients) who have experienced and conquered similar problems related to medical illness [1]. In addition to providing support, the role of group psychotherapy is to provide basic information, facilitate emotional expression, and teach coping skills [18, 19].

Group psychotherapy may offer benefits not available in individual settings, such as sharing a common experience and identity, a feeling of helping oneself by helping others, hopefulness fostered by observing how others have coped successfully, and a sense of belonging to a group [21]. Group participation helps decrease the sense of isolation and alienation, as the cancer patient and family can see that they are not alone in adjusting to the illness [1].

The topics for discussion in group psychotherapy are grief work, coping skills, mastery, cognitive reframing, and the reordering of priorities [21].

16.3.5 Self-Help Treatment

Most self-help support networks (e.g., Patient to Patient Program: Reach to Recovery, ostomy clubs) for cancer patients work closely with professional medical services, thereby offering social support as an adjunct to medical care. Volunteers help decrease patients' sense of alienation and isolation because of their unique knowledge and sensitivity, which comes with their shared experiences [1]. In particular, veteran patient volunteers facilitate coping in newly diagnosed patients by providing them with information, emotional support, and role models for successful adaptation and recovery [5].

16.3.6 Biopsychosocial Effects of Psychological and Behavioral Interventions

In group and individual therapy, patients reported less distress, higher self-esteem and self-image, less anxiety, and more self-control post-psychotherapy than pre-psychotherapy [22]. In addition, the level of satisfaction and compliance with therapy improved [23].

Mindfulness-based stress reduction (MBSR) programs are effective in decreasing mood disturbance and stress symptoms in patients with various cancer diagnoses and stages of illness [24].

16.3.7 Psychopharmacotherapy

Short-acting lorazepam is recommended in patients with hepatic cancer and anxiety. However, in terminal cancer patients with delirium, low-dose neuroleptics are preferred over benzodiazepine antianxiety agents, which may enhance confusion. Particularly in cancer patients with serious respiratory impairment, benzodiazepine antianxiety agents should not be used because of the risk of respiratory center suppression. However, antihistamines (e.g., diphenhydramine) can be used in these patients [1].

Mild or moderate depression often resolves spontaneously [25] with resolution of a precipitating stressor. However, patients with severe depression, such as major depressive disorder (MDD), may benefit significantly from pharmacotherapy, psychotherapy, or a combination of both [26]. Moreover, the combination of antidepressant and cognitive therapy may enhance long-term recovery from depression compared to cognitive therapy alone [27].

Tricyclic antidepressants are recommended in cancer patients experiencing anorexia and weight loss. In contrast, selective serotonin reuptake inhibitors (SSRIs) and venlafaxine tend to cause weight loss [28]. These drugs often cause side effects such as nausea and should be used with caution in patients with gastrointestinal cancer and those undergoing chemotherapy [29].

In particular, amitriptyline, which has a sedative action, is known to be effective in cancer patients with insomnia or emotional instability. This drug also helps relieve pain. For older patients, especially those with stomatitis caused by radiotherapy, it is better to use either trazodone or paroxetine, which have a sedative action but few anticholinergic effects [30].

SSRIs (e.g., paroxetine) can be effectively used in patients with cancer and depression, although they may cause nausea and vomiting [31]. Noradrenergic and specific serotonergic antidepressants (NaSSAs; e.g.,mirtazapine) may also be used in these patients [32], especially in those with poor appetite andinsomnia.

Case

A 59-year-old female patient was referred from the department of gynecology for psychiatric consultation at the outpatient clinic and then admitted to the department of psychiatry. At that time, she showed severe depression, agitation, suicidal rumination, and social withdrawal, and complained of a variety of somatic symptoms such as weakness, anorexia, insomnia, generalized ache, palpitation, and lethargy. 6 months earlier, she had undergone surgery for uterus cancer at the department of gynecology, after which she developed thrombosis in the left leg. She was admitted to the department of transplantation surgery for about 2 weeks, where she received medication such as 5 mg of warfarin (Coumadin), 300 mg of triflusal (Disgren), and 1 mg of lorazepam per day. She had been almost unable to walk for 1 month while suffering from the above symptoms.

The patient was diagnosed with major depressive disorder. Her husband took care of her all the time during admission. Amitriptyline 25 mg twice per day and ethyl loflazepate 1 mg before sleep were administered orally. She continued to complain of weakness and generalized ache, showing irritability for the first few days after admission. Around this time, when a psychiatric resident visited her, she showed signs of hopelessness, saying "Are you here to see me dying?" She was also anxious, saying, "It looks like my illness won't get better." The next day, however, her sleep improved, and she began to complain less frequently of her somatic symptoms. 8 days after hospitalization, she walked to another room to watch TV. The day after, she began to try to walk a little more, and her mood also improved. Thereafter, she continued to walk, had a better appetite, and started to have hopes for her improved physical condition. She once recalled with a bright facial expression, "I have enjoyed playing golf for a long time, but because I thought I could never play golf anymore when I was unable to walk, I lost my joy and meaning of life."

The patient was discharged 18 days after hospitalization, at which time she was able to walk by herself, felt better, and began to regain her physical strength. After eating out with her family, she said "I am considering traveling abroad in the near future."

This patient experienced damage to her self-esteem as she was weak and unable to walk because of thrombosis in the leg as a sequela of her cancer treatment. Thereafter, she was psychologically constricted and extremely limited in her own activities, showing hypersensitivity to minimal physical changes. Her frequently used cognitive coping mechanisms were extremism, catastrophism, and pessimism. However, increased physical activity as recommended by her therapist as well as improvements in sleep and in her depressed mood as a result of treatment with tricyclic antidepressants, along with her family's emotional support, especially her husband's devoted care, helped her gradually regain her self-confidence and self-respect.

16.4 Summary

1. To live with cancer is much more than adapting to the treatments and their side effects.
2. If psychiatric problems occur, psychiatric consultation should be considered.
3. The therapeutic approaches used in cancer patients are a combination of psychotherapeutic, behavioral, and psychopharmacologic techniques.
4. Psychotherapeutic approaches include cognitive therapy, family therapy, group therapy, and self-help treatment.
5. Behavioral approaches, such as muscle relaxation, systematic desensitization, cognitive distraction, and exercise intervention, are helpful for health-related quality of life.
6. A psychopharmacologic approach is effective against anxiety, depression, delirium, pain, nausea, vomiting, and insomnia.
7. An integrated approach that includes therapeutic techniques tailored to each individual's needs is strongly suggested.

References

1. Lesko, L. M., Massie, M. J., & Holland, J. C. (1987). Oncology. In A. Stoudemire & B. S. Fogel (Eds.), *Principles of medical psychiatry*. Grune & Stratton.

2. Wellisch, D. (1980). Psychosocial problems of cancer. In C. M. Haskell (Ed.), *Cancer treatment*. WB Saunders.
3. Worden, J. W. (1987). Cognitive therapy with cancer patients. In A. Freeman & V. Greenwood (Eds.), *Cognitive therapy: Applications in psychiatric and medical settings*. Human Science Press.
4. Cassem, N. H. (1991). The dying patient. In N. H. Cassem (Ed.), *MGH handbook of general hospital psychiatry. St.* Mosby Year Book.
5. Kaufman, E., & Micha, V. G. (1987). A model for psychotherapy with the good-prognosis cancer patient. *Psychosomatics, 28*, 540–547.
6. Marmor, J. (1979). Short-term dynamic psychotherapy. *The American Journal of Psychiatry, 136*, 149–155.
7. Bloom, J. R., Ross, R. D., & Burnell, G. (1978). The effect of social support on patient adjustment after breast surgery. *Patient Counselling and Health Education, 1*, 50–59.
8. Fiore, N. (1979). Fighting cancer: One patient's perspective. *The New England Journal of Medicine, 300*, 284–289.
9. Janis, E., & Mann, L. (1997). *Decision-making*. Free Press.
10. Spivack, G., Platt, J., & Schure, M. (1976). *The problem-solving approach to adjustment*. Jossey-Bass.
11. Benson, H. (1975). *The relaxation response*. Morrow.
12. Burish, T. G., & Lyles, J. N. (1981). Effectiveness of relaxation training in reducing adverse reactions to cancer chemotherapy. *Journal of Behavioral Medicine, 4*, 65–78.
13. Morrow, G. R., & Morrell, B. S. (1982). Behavioral treatment for the anticipatory nausea and vomiting induced by cancer chemotheray. *The New England Journal of Medicine, 306*, 1476–1480.
14. Redd, W. H., Andresen, G. V., & Minagawa, Y. (1982). Hypnotic control of anticipatory emesis in patients receiving cancer chemotherapy. *Journal of Consulting and Clinical Psychology, 50*, 14–19.
15. Mishra, S. I., Scherer, R. W., Snyder, C., et al. (2012). Exercise interventions on health-related quality of life for people with cancer during active treatment. *Cochrane Database of Systematic Reviews, 8*, CD008465. https://doi.org/10.1002/14651858.CD008465.pub2
16. Pfeffenbaum, G., Pasnau, R., & Jamison, K. (1977). A comprehensive program of psychosocial care for mastectomy patients. *International Journal of Psychiatry in Medicine, 8*, 65–71.
17. Schain, W. S. (1982). Sexual problems of patients with cancer. In V. T. Devita, S. Hellman, & S. A. Rosenberg (Eds.), *Cancer: Principles and practices of oncology*. JB Lippincott.
18. Fawzy, F. I., & Fawzy, N. W. (1998). Group therapy in the cancer setting. *Journal of Psychosomatic Research, 45*, 191–200.
19. Fawzy, F. I., & Fawzy, N. W. (1998). Psychoeducational interventions. In J. C. Holland (Ed.), *Textbook of psychooncology. Oxford Univ* (pp. 676–693). Press.
20. Spiegel D, Stein SL, Earhart TZ, et al. Group psychotherapy and the terminally ill. In: Chochinov H, Breitbart W, editors. The handbook of psychiatry in palliative medicine. Oxford Univ. Press; 2000. p. 241–251.
21. Breitbart, W. (2002). Spirituality and meaning in supportive care: Spirituality and meaning-centered group psychotherapy interventions in advanced cancer. *Support Care Cancer, 10*, 272–280.
22. Kubler-Ross, E. (1969). *On death and dying*. Macmillan.
23. Jerse, M. A., Whitman, H. H., & Gustafson, J. P. (1984). Cancer in adults. In H. B. Roback (Ed.), *Helping patients and their families cope with medical problems*. Jossey-Bass.
24. Carlson, L. E., Ursuliak, Z., Goodey, E., et al. (2001). The effects of a mindfulness meditation-based stress reduction program on mood and symptoms of stress in cancer outpatients: 6-moth follow-up. *Support Care Cancer, 9*, 112–123.
25. Williams, J. W., Barrett, J., Oxman, T., et al. (2000). Treatment of dysthymia and minor depression in primary care: A randomized controlled trial in older adults. *JAMA, 284*, 1519–1526.

26. Fann, J. R., Thomas-rich, A. M., Katon, W. J., et al. (2008). Major depression after breast cancer: A reivew of epidemiology and treatment. *General Hospital Psychiatry, 30*, 112–126.
27. Maguire, P., Hopwood, P., Tarrier, N., et al. (1985). Treatment of depression in cancer patients. *Acta Psychiatrica Scandinavica. Supplementum, 320*, 81–84.
28. Cunningham, L. A., Borison, R. L., & Carman, J. S. (1994). A comparison of venlafaxine, trazodone and placebo in major depression. *Journal of Clinical Psychopharmacology, 14*, 99–106.
29. Koh, K. B. (2011). *Stress and psychosomatic medicine.* Ilchokak.
30. Cunningham, L. A. (1994). Depression in the medically ill: Choosing an antidepressant. *The Journal of Clinical Psychiatry, 55*(Suppl AJ), 90–97.
31. Morrow, G. R., Hickok, J. T., Roscoe, J. A., et al. (2003). Differential effects of paroxetine on fatigue and depression: A randomized, double-blind trail from the University of Rochester Cancer Center Community Clinical Oncology Program. *Journal of Clinical Oncology, 21*, 4635–4641.
32. Thompson, D. S. (2000). Mirtazapine for the treatment of depression and nausea in breast and gynecological oncology. *Psychosomatics, 41*, 356–359.

Chapter 17
Specific Cancer

17.1 Breast Cancer

17.1.1 Psychosocial Issues

The times of the most frequent psychiatric referral of breast cancer patients are during initial treatment and during treatment of metastatic or recurrent disease at a radiation oncology clinic. There is a high incidence of major depressive disorder in the outpatient breast cancer population [1].

With breast cancer, a symbol of femininity may be compromised, and a woman's loss of a breast may interfere with her identity [2].

Suppression of anger is shown to be associated with a higher risk of breast malignancy [3]. On the other hand, anger is also associated with anxiety and can be frequently directed toward physicians, hospital staff, and family members [4].

17.1.2 Psychotherapeutic Interventions

Psychological interventions have been shown to facilitate psychological adaptation to breast cancer [5]. Psychological interventions include strategies to reduce stress, improve mood, alter health behaviors, and maintain adherence to cancer treatment and care [6].

As later illustrated in a case report, concerns regarding the loss of femininity can sometimes be overcome by the therapist helping the patient express her emotions and encouraging the husband to assist her without being confrontational [7].

In readjusting to normal life, diversions from the illness and self-validation (or relativizing) seem to be helpful during periods of convalescence and chemo/radiotherapy [8].

K. B. Koh, *Body, Mind and Spirituality*, https://doi.org/10.1007/978-3-032-11214-9_17

Anger as well as anxiety and depression should be appropriately managed, sometimes with the help of a psychiatrist. Effective psychotherapeutic treatment of depression has been found to affect the course of cancer.

Specifically, effective treatment of depression in cancer patients results in better adjustment to the illness, remitted symptoms, and reduced cost of care and may influence the disease course. Thus, the treatment of depression in these patients may be considered part of medical treatment [9].

17.1.3 Psychopharmacotherapy of Depression in Breast Cancer Patients

Selective serotonin reuptake inhibitors (SSRIs) (e.g., paroxetine) and noradrenergic and specific serotonergic antidepressants (NaSSAs) (e.g., mirtazapine) may be effective in improving depression [10, 11] and decreasing menopausal symptoms in breast cancer survivors [12, 13, 14, 15, 16, 17, 18]. In addition, the norepinephrine reuptake inhibitor reboxetine is known to be effective in breast cancer patients with major depressive disorder [19]. A study on the effects of the norepinephrine-dopamine reuptake inhibitor (NDRI) bupropion in patients with early-stage breast cancer receiving hormonal therapy after chemotherapy showed improvement in both sexual functioning and depression levels, as measured by the Beck Depression Inventory (BDI) [20]. In depressed patients with stomatitis following radiotherapy or chemotherapy, or urinary retention, antidepressants such as a tricyclic with low anticholinergic effect (e.g., nortriptyline) [21] and SSRIs are recommended.

However, clinicians should be conscious of the possibility that antidepressant efficacy will be lower in women taking estrogen antagonists, such as tamoxifen, because estrogen may serve as an adjunct to the treatment of depression in postmenopausal women [22].

17.1.4 Social Support for Breast Cancer Patients

Social support from a spouse, another intimate, or a physician, as well as actively seeking social support, has been shown to be related to higher natural killer (NK) cell activity in patients with stages I and II breast cancer [23].

In addition, social support for cancer patients has a significant influence on the course of their illness. For example, marital status and perceived social support were positively associated with survival in patients with breast cancer [24].

Case

A woman in her late 30 s with breast cancer who had undergone radical mastectomy became depressed, along with a perceived loss of femininity and loss of self-esteem caused by the mastectomy. After being discharged from the hospital, the patient was encouraged by her sister to see a psychiatrist. She said, "I can't tolerate living with only one breast" and complained of insomnia and a lack of interest in life. She also showed strong resentment and anger toward her husband, recalling that he had shown little concern about her situation and had returned home late at night a few times several months earlier. Accompanied by the patient, her husband said apprehensively, "My wife is trying to avoid sleeping in the same bed with me." During her sessions, the patient was allowed to vent her emotions, including anger toward her husband's negligence. Antidepressant (fluoxetine) and antianxiety (ethyl loflazepate) agents were administered twice daily. Her anger level was assessed using a hostility questionnaire. She recorded high scores on the anger subscale, saying "I seemed to get sick because I had a bad temper." Then, a variety of coping strategies were reviewed, including a few considered good for her situation. Through the application of the strategies, she began to introspectively search her inner self.

She found herself egotistic and self-centered, and she regretted getting into religion only externally but not internally. In addition, with her husband's understanding of the situation and his active assistance, the patient began to accept her own reality, to forgive her husband for mistreating her, and to regain her emotional stability and self-confidence.

The issue relevant to her loss of femininity was not directly confronted by the psychiatrist. Rather, she was encouraged to vent her anger and do her limited daily activities, while she would deal with issues surrounding her illness. Also, the therapist encouraged her husband to actively participate in the therapeutic session. Such measures as the therapist's effort and the husband's assistance helped the patient overcome her depression caused by the loss of femininity and anger toward her spouse and return to her routine activities.

17.1.5 Biopsychosocial Effects of Psychological Interventions

Behavioral changes, rather than immunity changes, have been shown to be influential in achieving weaker symptoms and higher functional status. Therefore, reducing distress is important in improving the health of patients with breast cancer [25]. Moreover, psychological adaptation in women with breast cancer can reduce anxiety and depressive mood and improve quality of life, which affects immune functions, such as increased production of the Th1 cytokine interleukin-2 (IL-2), interferon-gamma (IFN-γ), and tumor necrosis factor-α (TNF-α) [3].

17.2 Prostate Cancer

17.2.1 Psychosocial Issues

Prostate cancer has been a neglected area in psycho-oncology for decades [26]. However, as the incidence and prevalence of prostate cancer continue to rise, the number of men who need help and support to cope with the disease and treatment-related symptoms is increasing [27]. Contrary to other types of cancer, prostate cancer grows slowly; therefore, patients do nothing but monitor it closely. As a result of treatment, prostate cancer patients often experience specific problems such as micturition disturbance, incontinence, erectile disorders, and bowel problems, in addition to problems that generally accompany cancer, such as fatigue, anxiety, and pain [28].

The quality of life in patients with prostate cancer needs to be emphasized because treatments not only provide a good survival rate but also cause adverse side effects [29]. Patients with prostate cancer also need support in the psychological, informational, and daily living domains [30]. At prostate cancer diagnosis, low-to-moderate psychological distress is most common, with distress decreasing after treatment [31].

17.2.2 Psychosocial Interventions

Overall, psychosocial interventions, such as cognitive behavioral therapy, psychoeducational approaches, supportive therapy, and counseling, may have short-term beneficial effects on certain domains of well-being, as measured by the physical component of quality of life when compared with usual care [27]. Another prospective study found that men who were undecided regarding what treatment to receive experienced greater decision-related distress, although psychological and decision-related distress decreased over time regardless of treatment modality. Therefore, interventions for patients with prostate cancer should target decision-related distress and provide in-depth psychological support to those who experience ongoing difficulties [31].

17.2.3 Social Support for Prostate Cancer Patients

Men with prostate cancer experience physical, psychological, healthcare system-related, and sexual issues [32]. Therefore, therapeutic team members should focus on the physical, psychological, social, and sexual needs of cancer patients [33].

17.2.4 Psychopharmacotherapy of Depression in Prostate Cancer Patients

Various antidepressants are used to treat patients with prostate cancer and depression. In particular, venlafaxine [34] and paroxetine [35] have proven effective in reducing hot flashes, the most common complaint reported by men undergoing androgen suppression treatment for prostate cancer.

A case example of prostate cancer is illustrated in Chap. 6, which shows the importance of spiritual approaches, such as prayer and access to Bible verses, immediately before procedures undertaken to assess whether the cancer spread to the bones as well as surgical operations.

17.3 Summary

1. Breast cancer patients with persistent concerns regarding body image, sexual desire, and sexual function should be referred to professionals.
2. Clinicians should be conscious of the possibility that antidepressant efficacy will be lower in women taking an estrogen antagonist, such as tamoxifen.
3. The quality of life in prostate cancer patients needs to be emphasized because treatments not only provide a good survival rate but also cause adverse side effects.
4. Prostate cancer patients need support in psychological, informational, and daily living domains.
5. A variety of antidepressants can be used in depressed patients with breast or prostate cancer.

References

1. Pendlebury, S. C., & Snars, J. (1996). Role of a psychiatry liaison clinic in the management of breast cancer. *Australasian Radiology, 40*, 283–286.
2. Daune, F. (1995). Psychological aspects of breast cancer. *Revue Médicale de Bruxelles, 16*, 245–247.
3. Blomberg, B. B., Alvarez, J. P., Diaz, A., et al. (2009). Psychosocial adaptation and cellular immunity in breast cancer patients in the weeks after surgery: An exploratory study. *Journal of Psychosomatic Research, 67*, 369–376.
4. Peck, A. (1972). Emotional reactions to having cancer. *Radium Ther Nucl Med, 114*, 591–599.
5. McGregor, B. A., & Antoni, M. H. (2009). Psychological intervention and health outcomes among women treated for breast cancer: A review of stress pathways and biological mediators. *Brain, Behavior, and Immunity, 23*, 159–166.
6. Andersen, B. L., Yang, H. C., Farrar, W. B., et al. (2008). Psychologic intervention improves survival for breast cancer patients: A randomized clinical trial. *Cancer, 113*, 3450–3458.

7. Koh, K. B. (2013). Psychosocial aspects of breast cancer: Focus on interventions. In K. B. Koh (Ed.), *Somatization and psychosomatic symptoms*. Springer.
8. Heim, E., Augustiny, K. F., Schaffner, L., et al. (1993). Coping with breast cancer over time and situation. *Journal of Psychosomatic Research, 37*, 523–542.
9. Spiegel, D. (1996). Cancer and depression. *The British Journal of Psychiatry, 30*(Suppl), 109–116.
10. Morrow, G. R., Hickok, J. T., Roscoe, J. A., et al. (2003). Differential effects of paroxetine on fatigue and depression: A randomized, double-blind trail from the University of Rochester Cancer Center Community Clinical Oncology Program. *Journal of Clinical Oncology, 21*, 4635–4641.
11. Thompson, D. S. (2000). Mirtazapine for the treatment of depression and nausea in breast and gynecological oncology. *Psychosomatics, 41*, 356–359.
12. Gordon, P. R., Kerwin, J. P., Boesen, K. G., et al. (2006). Sertraline to treat hot flashes: A a randomized controlled, double-blind, crossover trial in a general population. *Menopause, 13*, 568–575.
13. Kimmick, G. G., Lovato, J., McQuellon, R., et al. (2006). Randomized, double-blind, placebo-controlled, crossover study of sertraline (Zoloft) for the treatment of hot flashes in women with early stage breast cancer taking tamoxifen. *The Breast Journal, 12*, 114–122.
14. Loprinzi, C. L., Kugler, J. W., Sloan, J. A., et al. (2000). Venlafaxine in management of hot flashes in survivors of breast cancer: A randomized controlled trial. *Lancet, 356*, 2059–2063.
15. Loprinzi, C. L., Sloan, J. A., Perez, E. A., et al. (2002). Phase III evaluation of fluoxetine for treatment of hot flashes. *Journal of Clinical Oncology, 20*, 1578–1583.
16. Soares, C. N., Poitras, J. R., Prouty, J., et al. (2003). Efficacy of citalopram as a monotherapy or as an adjunctive treatment to estrogen therapy for perimenopausal and postmenopausal women with depression and vasomotor symptoms. *The Journal of Clinical Psychiatry, 64*, 473–479.
17. Stearns, V., Beebe, K. L., Iyengar, M., et al. (2003). Paroxetine controlled release in the treatment of menopausal hot flashes: A randomized controlled trial. *JAMA, 289*, 2827–2834.
18. Stearns, V., Issacs, C., Rowland, J., et al. (2000). A pilot trial assessing the efficacy of paroxetine hydrochloride (Paxil) in controlling hot flashes in breast cancer survivors. *Annals of Oncology, 11*, 17–22.
19. Grassi, L., Biancosino, B., Marmai, L., et al. (2004). Effect of reboxetine on major depressive disorder in breast cancer patients: An open-label study. *The Journal of Clinical Psychiatry, 65*, 515–520.
20. Mathias, C., Cardeal Mendes, C. M., Ponde de Sena, E., et al. (2006). An open-label, fixed-dose study of bupropion effect on sexual function scores in women treated for breast cancer. *Annals of Oncology, 17*, 1792–1796.
21. Lesko, L. M., Massie, M. J., & Holland, J. C. (1987). Oncology. In A. Stoudemire & B. S. Fogel (Eds.), *Principles of medical psychiatry*. Grune & Stratton.
22. Fann, J. R., Thomas-rich, A. M., Katon, W. J., et al. (2008). Major depression after breast cancer: A reivew of epidemiology and treatment. *General Hospital Psychiatry, 30*, 112–126.
23. Levy, S. M., Herberman, R. B., Whiteside, T., et al. (1990). Perceived social support and tumor-estrogen/progesterone receptor status as predictors of natural killer cell activity in breast cancer patients. *Psychosomatic Medicine, 52*, 73–85.
24. Spiegel, D., & Kato, P. M. (1996). Psychosocial influences on cancer incidence and progression. *Harvard Rev Psychiatry, 4*, 10–26.
25. Andersen, B. L., Golden-Kreutz, D., Emery, C. F., et al. (2007). Distress reduction from a psychological intervention contributes to improved health for cancer patients. *Brain, Behavior, and Immunity, 21*, 953–961.
26. Visser, A., & van Andel, G. (2003). Psychosocial and educational aspects in prostate cancer patients. *Patient Education and Counseling, 49*, 203–206.
27. Parahoo, K., McDonough, S., McCaughan, E., et al. (2013). Psychosocial interventions for men with prostate cancer. *Cochrane Database of Systematic Reviews, 12*, CD008529. https://doi.org/10.1002/14651858.CC008529.pub3

28. Voerman, B., Fischer, M., Visser, A., et al. (2004). Prostate cancer: A review of the literature on psychosocial problems and psychosocial interventions. *Gedrag en Gezondh: Tijdschr Psychol Gezondh, 32*, 251–270.
29. van Andel, G., Bottemley, A., Fossa, S. D., et al. (2008). An international field study of the EORTC QLQ-PR25: A questionnaire for assessing the health-related quality of life of patients with prostate cancer. *European J Cancer, 44*, 2418–2424.
30. Sanson-Fisher, R., Girgis, A., Boyes, A., et al. (2000). The unmet supportive care needs of patients with cancer. *Cancer, 88*, 226–237.
31. Steginga, S. K., Occhipinti, S., Gardiner, R. A., et al. (2004). Prospective study of men's psychological and decision-related adjustment after treatment for localized prostate cancer. *Urol, 63*, 751–756.
32. Daeter, L. V., & A, Van der Hooft-Lemans T. (2012). *Determinants of seeking psychosocial care in Dutch men with prostate cancer*. Master thesis. Report De Vruchtenburg.
33. Visser, A. (2013). Cancer in a psychosomatic perspective. In K. B. Koh (Ed.), *Somatization and psychosomatic symptoms*. Springer.
34. Irani, J., Salomon, L., Oba, R., et al. (2010). Efficacy of venlafaxine, medroxyprogesterone acetate, and cyproterone acetate for the treatment of vasomotor hot flushes in men taking gonadotropin-releasing hormone analogues for prostate cancer: A double-blind, randomized trial. *The Lancet Oncology, 11*, 147–154.
35. Naoe, M., Ogawa, Y., Shichijo, T., et al. (2006). Pilot evaluation of serotonin reuptake inhibitor antidepressants in hot flash patients under androgen-deprivation therapy for prostate cancer. *Prostate Cancer and Prostatic Diseases, 9*, 275–278.

Epilogue: My Personal Experience of Spirituality

I thank God for giving me the inspiration to write this book. With the completion of this work, I would like to share my personal experience of spirituality and some inspiring Bible verses that have enhanced my resilience. Finally, my poem "Prayer for an eraser" is included here.

Episodes of My Spiritual Experience

Rain of Love

"Your Father in heaven causes his sun to rise on the evil and the good, and sends rain on the righteous and the unrighteous" (Matthew 5:45). I was deeply moved when I read this Bible verse. Regardless of whether one is good or evil, God sends rain to all. Oh, this is God's love! The rain I once regarded thoughtlessly became, to me, the rain of love.

"Love your enemies and pray for those who persecute you" (Matthew 5:44). This Bible verse is also related to the one quoted above. Although it is difficult for us to follow what it says, we cannot help but accept that there is no other way to make peace in our life.

Two Crosses

One day, more than 20 years ago, early one morning I saw two dazzling white crosses (one square and the other rectangular) reflected on the windows of an apartment building opposite mine.

At the time, I thought they might be telling me to believe in God more firmly. However, their meaning has long remained a mystery.

K. B. Koh, *Body, Mind and Spirituality*, https://doi.org/10.1007/978-3-032-11214-9

After more than 10 years, this event came to mind again. I realized that one cross represented my soul, and the other, another soul.

I Dream of a Miracle That Debt Would Turn to Light

In my mid-50s, an episode that occurred during my high school days suddenly came to mind on my way home from the subway station. It occurred to me that I had once lived as a debtor and did not try to pay my debt.

I long suffered from intolerable abdominal pain. Thus, I promised to do as God would want me to in order to cure my illness. However, I forgot my promise after I recovered fully from the illness. A few years before my retirement, I underwent a gastroscopy examination, which revealed scarring from a duodenal ulcer.

Following this event, I really changed. To repay my debt, I decided to do something for God. I began to participate in worship dramas at church. I also attempted to write spiritual poems and books to comfort others' souls. I liked to talk to the spirit and dreamed of a miracle where debt would be transformed into light.

Enthralling Bible Verses Enhancing Resilience

The following Bible verses may help increase resilience during difficult times and when dealing with serious health conditions.

Ephesians

2:8 For it is by grace you have been saved, through faith—and this not from yourselves, it is the gift of God—

2:9 not works, so that no one can boast.

2:10 For we are God's workmanship, created in Jesus Christ to do good works, which God prepared in advance for us to do.

Meditation: I realized that my belief was not chosen by me, but by grace, and that I have been saved by the belief. Henceforth, we will have to do good in Jesus Christ. Moreover, doing so cannot be our boast.

John

15:15 I no longer call you servants, because a servant does not know his master's business. Instead, I have called you friends, for everything that I learned from my Father I have made known to you.

15:16 You did not choose me, but I chose you and appointed you to go and bear fruit—fruit that will last. Then the Father will give you whatever you ask in my name.

15:17 This is my command: Love each other.

Meditation: God, who chose me to bear fruit, gives whatever I ask in the name of Jesus. He aims to make us love each other. I realize how great his love is.

Thessalonians

5:15 Make sure that nobody pays back wrong for wrong, but always try to be kind to each other and everyone else;

5:16 Be joyful always;

5:17 Pray continually;

5:18 Give thanks in all circumstances, for this is God's will for you in Jesus Christ.

Meditation: I used to resent someone who hurt me. I hated them. Let me be kind to them, with the help of the Holy Spirit. Our life is a gift. God wants us to live together peacefully. Please help me live in joy, thanksgiving, and prayer in Jesus Christ. Thank you for letting me know that living so is God's will.

John

14:6 I am the way and the truth and the life. No one comes to the Father except through me.

8:32 Then you will know the truth, and the truth will set you free.

Meditation: This verse makes us aware that Jesus is the way and the truth, not the knowledge and wisdom of the world. His word is truth, and by believing in his words, we will be freed from being servants of sins.

Philippians

4:12 I know what it is to be in need, and I know what it is to have plenty. I have learned the secret of being content in any and every situation, whether well fed or hungry, whether living in plenty or in want.

4:13 I can do everything through him who gives me strength.

Meditation: If we always live in Jesus regardless of whether we have difficulties, it reminds us that we can feel peace, joy, and self-contentment in our life. Please forgive us for seeking God's help only in times of difficulty. Please let us believe that the power of spirituality will help us overcome any difficulties we are unable to overcome ourselves.

Matthew

11:28 Come to me, all you who are weary and burdened, and I will give you rest.

11:29 Take my yoke upon you and learn from me, for I am gentle and humble in heart, and you will find rest for your souls.

11:30 For my yoke is easy and my burden is light.

Meditation: I have always been overwhelmed by a great deal of burden. I could not take the load off my mind because of greed for things in the world, even though they are very heavy. The more I have, the more I try to have. I realized that it is my sin that distances me from God. Let me surrender any greed that is beyond my reach and learn gentleness and humility from Jesus so that I may lighten the burden of life and experience true rest and peace of mind.

Matthew

4:3 If you are the son of God, tell these stones to become bread.

4:4 Man does not live on bread alone, but on every word that comes from the mouth of God.

Meditation: Jesus' response to Satan's temptation in the wilderness is deeply moving. We reflect on ourselves, who are vulnerable to the temptations of material things and have sinned a great deal. Please help us feel that the word of God is more precious than material things.

Isaiah

41:10 Do not fear, for I am with you; do not be dismayed, for I am your God. I will strengthen you and help you; I will uphold you with my righteous right hand.

Meditation: I underwent an operation for prostate cancer approximately a year and a half ago. I noticed this Bible verse on the upper part of the entrance to the operating room and on the ceiling of the room. I no longer felt lonely and remained calm during the operation. Sometimes, we have the opportunity to be completely dependent on God because we are helpless when facing difficult situations or dealing with serious health conditions. He can give us strength and raise us up.

Rome

5:1 Therefore, since we have been justified through faith, we have peace with God through our Lord Jesus Christ,

5:2 through whom we have gained access by faith into this grace in which we now stand. And we rejoice in the hope of the glory of God.

5:3 Not only so, but we also rejoice in our sufferings, because we know that suffering produces perseverance;

5:4 perseverance, character; and character, hope.

Meditation: When unhappy events occur, people, even when they are Christians, are likely to resent God. A middle-aged woman who was admitted to a hospital after a head injury due to a traffic accident resented God and asked in an angry voice, "Why did this terrible thing happen to me, even though I believed in God fervently?"

Whenever we face difficulties in life, it is important to reflect on what we must accept—things we cannot change. This encourages constructive actions to direct our lives positively with the help of God, even though it is not easy to bring change into our lives.

Looking back, we realize that our difficult and painful past experiences have been stimuli for growth.

Galatians

6:9 Let us not become weary in doing good, for at the proper time we will reap a harvest if we do not give up.

Meditation: We may feel disappointed and frustrated while doing good in Jesus Christ. This may be because we face obstacles, such as poor resources (e.g., financial problems, lack of human resources) and interpersonal relationships. However, the verse, “if we endure without giving up, we will bear fruit someday” give us strength.

Psalms

18:1 I love you, O Lord, my strength

18:2 The Lord is my rock, my fortress and my deliverer;
my God is my rock, in whom I take refuge.
He is my shield and the horn of my salvation, my stronghold.

18:6 In my distress I called to the Lord;

I cried to my God for help.
From his temple he heard my voice;
my cry came before him, into his ears.

Meditation: The God we believe in is love and strength. He is the rock in whom we can take refuge. He is the shield and deliverer. As David said, let us cry to God for help when we are in distress. He hears our voice and will help us someday.

Acts

20:35 In everything I did, I showed you that by this kind of hard work we must help the weak, remembering the words the Lord Jesus himself said: it is more blessed to give than to receive.

Meditation: After listening to a Western doctor and missionary from Korea, an American businessman proposed a large sum of money for his project (building a general hospital in Korea for the first time). When the missionary (Dr. Evison) said, "Thank you so much," the businessman (Mr. Severance) responded, "It is more joyful to give than to receive." This is how the first Western hospital (Severance Hospital, Yonsei University) was established in Korea. I once again realized that "the word of God is living and active" (Hebrews 4:12).

Poem for Our Soul

This is a poem by the author KB Koh

Prayer for an Eraser

> There's something unforgotten
> and too painful to say.
>
> To erase the name
> that has left a sinkhole
> in my heart
>
> I try as I might,
> but it's not erased.
>
> What do I do?
>
> Toward heaven,
> I have no choice but
> to put my hands together and say,
> "Please give me an eraser."

Index

K. B. Koh, *Body, Mind and Spirituality*, https://doi.org/10.1007/978-3-032-11214-9

C

D

E

T

U

V

W

MIX
Papier aus verantwortungsvollen Quellen
Paper from responsible sources
FSC® C105338

If you have any concerns about our products,
you can contact us on
ProductSafety@springernature.com

In case Publisher is established outside the EU,
the EU authorized representative is:
Springer Nature Customer Service Center GmbH
Europaplatz 3, 69115 Heidelberg, Germany

Printed by Libri Plureos GmbH
in Hamburg, Germany